D1785537

THE ART OF THE

KAMA SUTRA

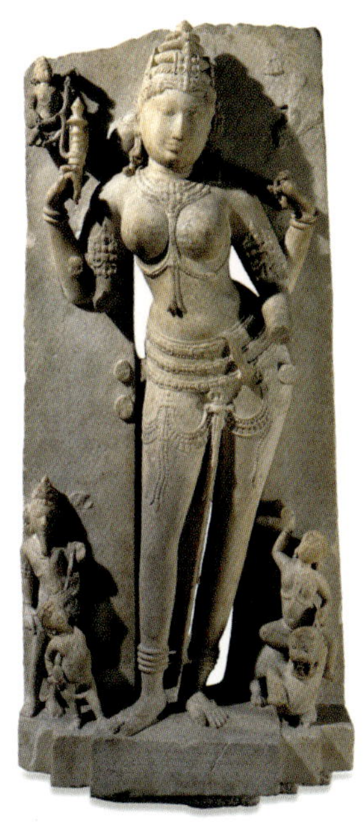

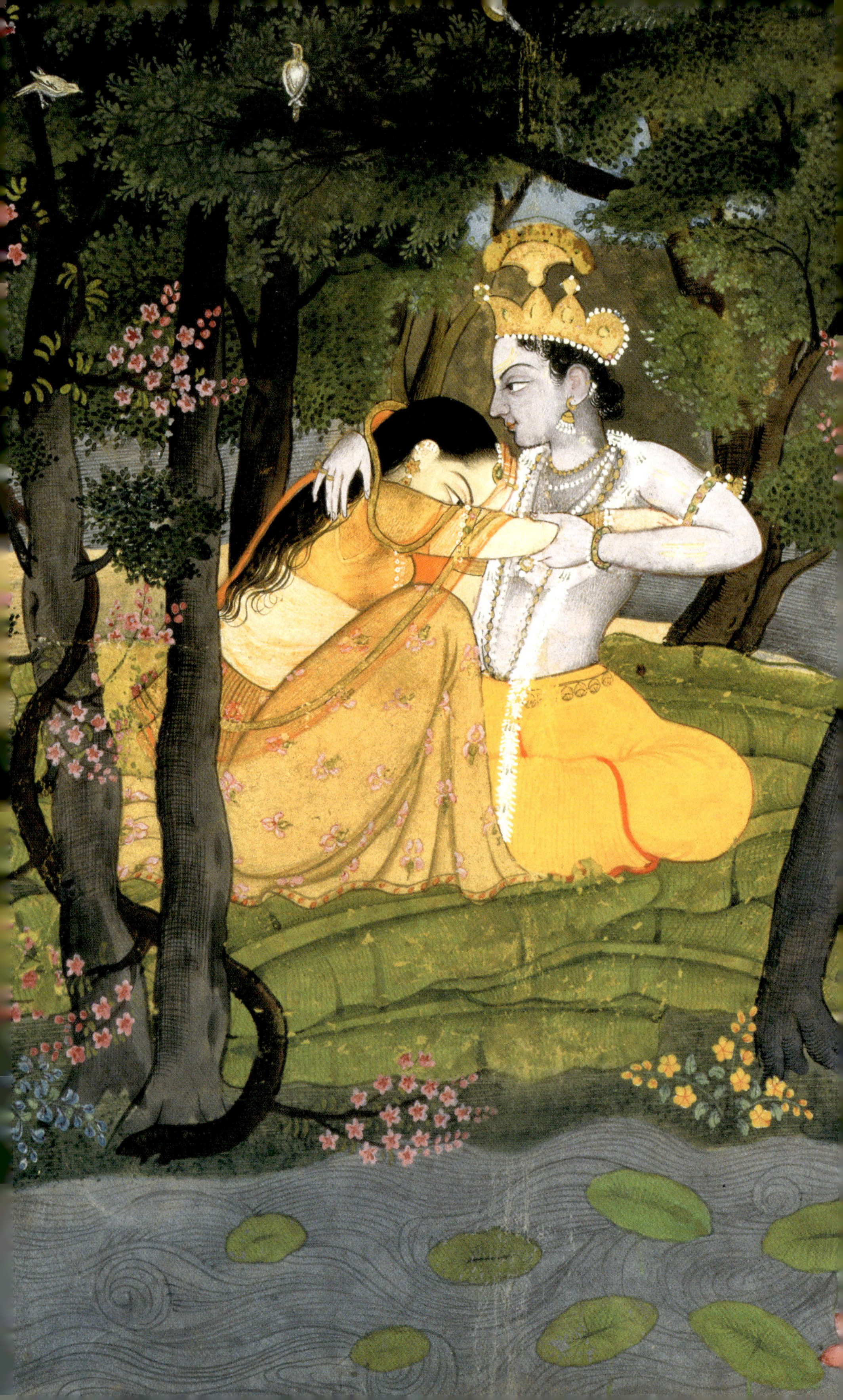

THE ART OF THE KAMA SUTRA

MALLANAGA VATSYAYANA

AN EDITED VERSION OF THE ORIGINAL TRANSLATION BY SIR RICHARD BURTON AND F.F. ARBUTHNOT

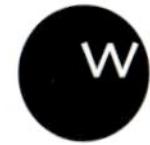

WATKINS PUBLISHING
LONDON

The Art of the Kama Sutra
Mallanaga Vatsyayana

First published in the United Kingdom and Ireland in 2011 by
Watkins Publishing, an imprint of Duncan Baird Publishers Ltd
Sixth Floor, Castle House
75–76 Wells Street
London W1T 3QH

Conceived, created and designed by Duncan Baird Publishers

Managing Editor: Christopher Westhorp
Managing Designer: Suzanne Tuhrim
Picture Research: Susannah Stone

British Library Cataloguing-in-Publication Data:
A CIP record for this book is available from the British Library

ISBN: 978-1-907486-30-2

10 9 8 7 6 5 4 3 2 1

Typeset in Adobe Garamond and Linotype Zapfino
Colour reproduction by Colourscan
Printed in Singapore by Imago

Note:
This translation is a modernized version of the one produced originally by Sir Richard Burton and F.F. Arbuthnot for their 1885 edition. Arranged here into *sutras*, the text has been amended modestly for a modern audience.

Contents

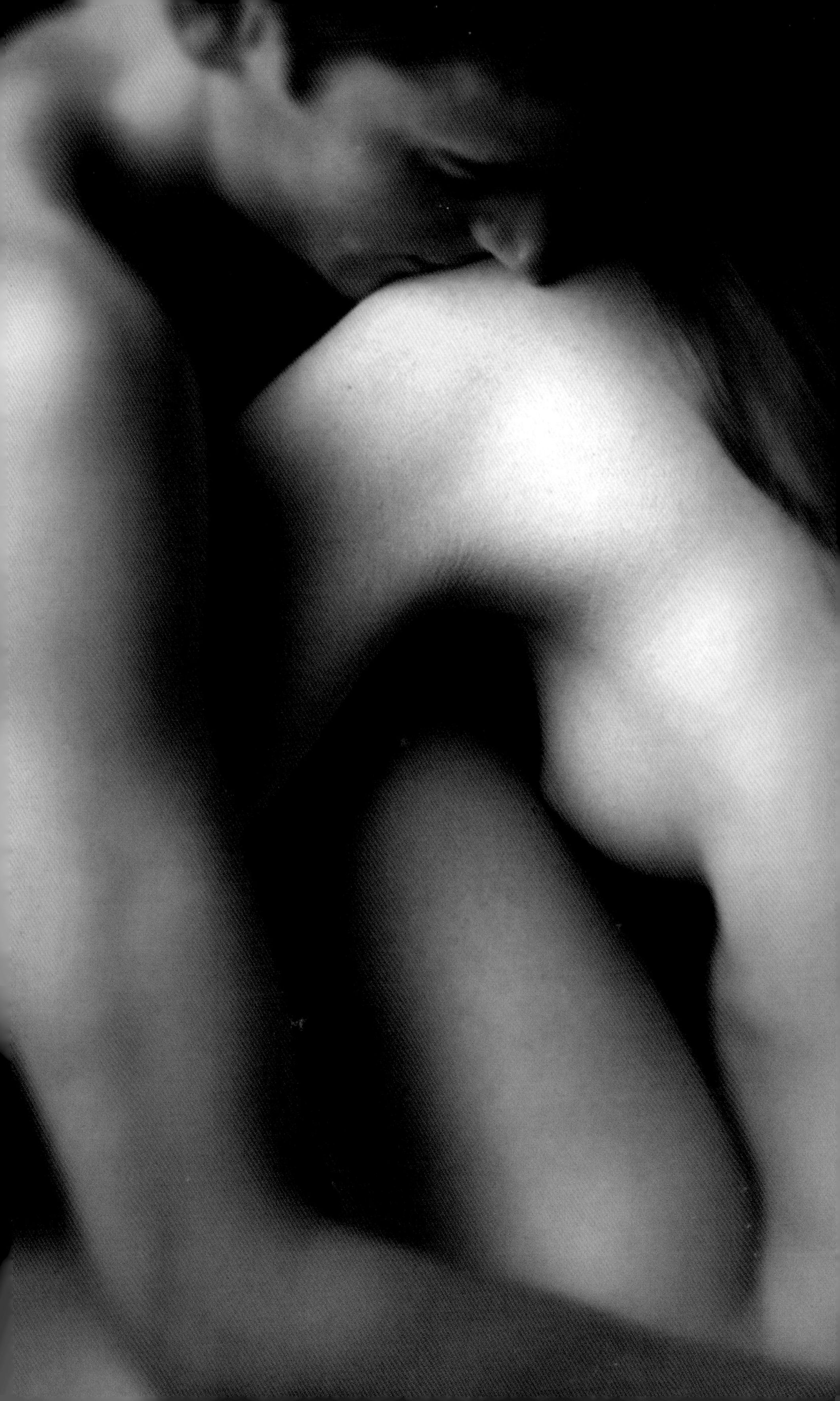

Preface

In the literature of all countries there will be found a certain number of works dealing with love. Everywhere the subject is treated differently, and from various points of view. In the present publication it is proposed to give a complete translation of what is considered the standard work on love in Sanskrit literature, and which is called the *Vatsyayana Kama Sutra*, or "Aphorisms on Love" by Vatsyayana.

While the introduction will deal with the evidence concerning the date of the writing, and the commentaries written upon it, the chapters following the introduction will give a translation of the work itself. It is, however, advisable to furnish here a brief analysis of works of the same nature, prepared by authors who lived and wrote years after Vatsyayana had passed away, but who still considered him as the great authority, and always quoted him as the chief guide to Hindu erotic literature.

Besides the treatise of Vatsyayana the following works on the same subject are procurable in India: the *Ratirahasya*, or "Secrets of Love"; the *Panchasakya*, or "Five Arrows"; the *Smara Pradipa*, or "Light of Love"; the *Ratimanjari*, or "Garland of Love"; the *Rasmanjari*, or "Sprout of Love"; the *Ananga Ranga*, or "Stage of Love", also called *Kamaledhiplava*, or "Boat in the Ocean of Love".

The author of the "Secrets of Love" was a poet named Kukkoka. He composed his work to please one Venudutta, who was perhaps a king. When writing his own name at the end of each chapter he calls himself "Siddha patiya pandita", an ingenious man among learned men. The work was translated into Hindi years ago, and the author's name was written as Koka. And as the same name crept into all the translations into other languages in India, the book became generally known as, and the subject was popularly called, the *Koka Shastra*, or "Doctrines of Koka", which is identical with the *Kama Shastra*, or "Doctrines of Love", and the names *Koka Shastra* and *Kama Shastra* are used indiscriminately.

The work contains nearly 800 verses, and is divided into ten chapters, which are called *pachivedas*. Some of the things discussed in this work are not to be found in the *Vatsyayana*, such as the four classes of women – the Padmini, Chitrini, Shankini and Hastini – or the enumeration of the days and hours on which the women of the different classes become subject to love. The author adds that he wrote these things based on the opinions of Gonikaputra and Nandikeshwara, both of whom are mentioned by Vatsyayana, but whose works have been lost. It is difficult to give any idea as to the year in which the *Koka Shastra* was composed. It is only to be presumed that it was written after the *Vatsyayana*, and previous to the other surviving works on this subject. Vatsyayana names ten authors on the subject, all of whose writings he had consulted, but none of which is extant, and he does not mention Kukkoka's work. This suggests Kukkoka wrote after Vatsyayana, otherwise Vatsyayana would assuredly have mentioned him.

The author of the "Five Arrows" was one Jyotirisha. He says that he composed the work after reflecting on the aphorisms of love as revealed by the gods, and studying the opinions of Gonikaputra, Muladeva, Babhravya, Ramtideva, Nundikeshwara and Kshemandra. It is impossible to say whether he had perused all the writings of these authors, or had only heard about them; anyhow, none of them appears to exist now. The work contains nearly 600 verses, and is divided into five chapters, called *sayakas* or "arrows".

The author of the "Light of Love" was the poet Gunakara, the son of Vechapati. The book contains 400 verses, and gives only a short account of the doctrines of love, dealing more with other matters.

The "Garland of Love" is the work of the famous poet Jayadeva, who said about himself that he is a writer on all subjects. This treatise is, however, very short, containing only 125 verses.

The author of the "Sprout of Love" was a poet called Bhanudatta. It appears from the last verse of the manuscript that he was a resident of the province of Tirhoot, and son of a Brahmin named Ganeshwar. The work, written in Sanskrit, describes different classes of men and women. It contains three chapters, and its date cannot be ascertained.

The "Stage of Love" was composed by the poet Kullianmull, for the amusement of Ladkhan, the son of Ahmed Lodi, and supposed to have been a relation or connection of the house of Lodi. The work was written in the fifteenth or sixteenth century. It contains ten chapters, and has been translated into English but only six copies were printed for private circulation. This is supposed to be the latest of the Sanskrit works on the subject of love, and the ideas in it were evidently taken from previous writings of the same nature.

The contents of these works are in themselves a literary curiosity. There is to be found in Sanskrit poetry and drama contains a certain amount of sentiment and romance, but the subject of physical love is treated in a plain, simple, matter-of-fact sort of way. Men and women are classified and divided in the same way as the animal world. Just as Venus was the Western archetype of female beauty, the Padmini or "Lotus woman" was described by Hindus as the perfection of femininity, for example in the following account:

"She in whom the following signs and symptoms appear is called a Padmini. Her face is pleasing as the full moon; her body, well clothed with flesh, is soft as the mustard flower, her skin is fine, tender and fair as the yellow lotus, never dark coloured. Her eyes are bright and beautiful as the orbs of the fawn, well cut, and with reddish corners. Her bosom is hard, full and high; she has a good neck; her nose is straight and lovely, and three folds or wrinkles cross her middle – about the umbilical region. Her *yoni* resembles the opening lotus bud, and her love seed (*kama salila*) is perfumed like the lily that has newly burst. She walks with swan-like gait, and her voice is low and musical as the note of the kokila bird. She delights in white raiments, in fine jewels, and in rich dresses. She eats little, sleeps lightly, and being as respectful and religious as she is clever and courteous, she is ever anxious to worship the gods, and to enjoy the conversation of Brahmins. Such, then, is the Padmini or Lotus woman."

There are also to be found detailed descriptions of the *chitrini* or "Art woman", the *shankhini* or "Conch woman", and the *hastini* or "Elephant woman", their days of enjoyment, their seats of passion, the manner in which they should be manipulated and treated in sexual intercourse, along with the characteristics of the men and women of the various regions of India.

One work in English somewhat similar to these is *Kalogynomia, or, The laws of female beauty: being the elementary principles of that science*, by T. Bell, M.D., and printed in London in 1821. It deals with beauty, love, sexual intercourse, the laws regulating that intercourse, monogamy and polygamy, prostitution, infidelity, and ends with a *catalogue raisonnée* of the defects of female beauty. Other works in English also enter into details of private and domestic life: *The Elements of Social Science, or Physical, Sexual and Natural Religion*, by a Doctor of Medicine, London, 1880, and *Every Woman's Book*, by Dr Waters, 1826. These works contain details seldom before published, and which ought to be understood by all philanthropists and benefactors of society.

After a perusal of the Hindu work, and of the English books mentioned, the reader will understand the subject of love, at all events from a materialistic, realistic and practical point of view. If all science is founded more or less on a stratum of facts, there can be no harm in making known to mankind matters intimately connected with their private, domestic and social life.

Alas! complete ignorance of them has wrecked many a man and woman, while a little knowledge of a subject generally ignored by the masses would have enabled many people to have understood things which they believed to be quite incomprehensible, or which were not thought worthy of their consideration.

Introduction

It may be interesting to some persons to learn how it came about that Vatsyayana was first brought to light and translated into English. A reading of the *Ananga Ranga*, or the "Stage of Love", revealed numerous references to one Vatsya: the sage Vatsya was of this opinion, or of that opinion; the sage Vatsya said this, and so on. Naturally, questions were asked who the sage was, and the pundits replied that Vatsya was the author of the standard work on love in Sanskrit literature, that no Sanskrit library was complete without his work, and that it was most difficult now to obtain in its entirety. The manuscript in Bombay was defective, and so the pundits wrote to Benares, Calcutta and Jeypoor for copies from Sanskrit libraries in those places. Copies having been obtained, they were then compared, and with the aid of a commentary called *Jayamangla* a revised copy of the manuscript was prepared, and from this copy the English translation was made. The following is the certificate of the chief pundit:

"The accompanying manuscript is corrected by me after comparing four different copies of the work. I had the assistance of a commentary called *Jayamangla* for correcting the portion in the first five parts, but found great difficulty in correcting the remaining portion, because, with the exception of one copy thereof which was tolerably correct, all the other copies I had were far too incorrect. However, I took that portion as correct in which the majority of the copies agreed with each other."

The "Aphorisms on Love" by Vatsyayana contains about 1,250 *sloka*s, or verses, and is divided into parts, parts into chapters, and chapters into paragraphs. The whole consists of seven parts, thirty-six chapters and sixty-four paragraphs. Hardly anything is known about the author. His real name is supposed to be Mallinaga or Mrillana, Vatsyayana being his family name. At the close of the work this is what he writes about himself:

"After reading and considering the works of Babhravya and other ancient authors, and thinking over the meaning of the rules given by them, this treatise was composed, according to the precepts of the Holy Writ, for the benefit of the world, by Vatsyayana, while leading the life of a religious student at Benares, and wholly engaged in the contemplation of the Deity. This work is not to be used merely as an instrument for satisfying our desires. A person acquainted with the true principles of this science, who preserves his Dharma (virtue or religious merit), his Artha (worldly wealth) and his Kama (pleasure or sensual gratification), and who has regard to the customs of the people, is sure to obtain the mastery over his senses. In short, an intelligent and knowing person attending to Dharma and Artha and also to Kama, without becoming the slave of his passions, will obtain success in everything that he may do."

It is impossible to fix the exact date either of the life of Vatsyayana or of his work. It is supposed that he must have lived between the first and sixth century of the Common Era, on the following grounds. He mentions that Satakarni Satavahana, a king of Kuntal, killed Malayavati his wife with an instrument called a *kartari* by striking her in the passion of love, and Vatsya quotes this case to warn people of the danger arising from some old customs of striking women when under the influence of this passion (see page 83). This king is believed to have reigned during the first century CE, and consequently Vatsya must have lived after him. On the other hand, Virahamihira, in the eighteenth chapter of his *Brihatsanhita*, deals with the science of love and appears to have borrowed largely from Vatsyayana. Virahamihira is said to have lived during the sixth century CE, and as Vatsya must have written his works previously, not earlier than the first century CE and not later than the sixth century must be the approximate date of his existence.

Only two commentaries on the "Aphorisms on Love" have been found. One called *Jayamangla*, or *Sutrabashya*, and the other *Sutra vritti*. The date of the *Jayamangla* is fixed between the tenth and thirteenth centuries CE, because the example of the sixty-four arts is taken from the *Kavyaprakasha*, which was written in about the tenth century. Again, the copy of the commentary procured was a transcript of a manuscript which once had a place in the library of a Chaulukyan king named Vishaladeva. It is well known that this king ruled in Gujarat from 1244 to 1262. The date, therefore, of the commentary is taken to be not earlier than the tenth and not later than the thirteenth century. The author of it is supposed to be one Yashodhara, the name given him by his preceptor being Indrapada. He seems to have written it during the time of affliction caused by his separation from a clever and shrewd woman, at least that is what he himself says at the end of each chapter. It is presumed that he called his work after the name of his absent mistress, or the word may have some connection with the meaning of her name.

This commentary was most useful in explaining the true meaning of Vatsyayana, for the commentator appears to have had a considerable knowledge of the times of the older author, and gives in some places very detailed information. This cannot be said of the other commentary, called *Sutra vritti*, which was written in about 1789 by Narsing Shastri, a pupil of a Sarveshwar Shastri; the latter was a descendant of Bhaskur, and so also was our author, for at the conclusion of every part he calls himself Bhaskur Narsing Shastri. He was induced to write the work by order of the learned Raja Vrijalala, while he was residing in Benares (modern Varanasi in Uttar Pradesh), but as to the merits of this commentary it does not deserve much commendation. In many cases the writer does not appear to have understood the meaning of the original author, and has changed the text in many places to fit in with his own explanations.

A complete translation of the original work now follows. It has been prepared in complete accordance with the text of the manuscript.

The Kama Sutra

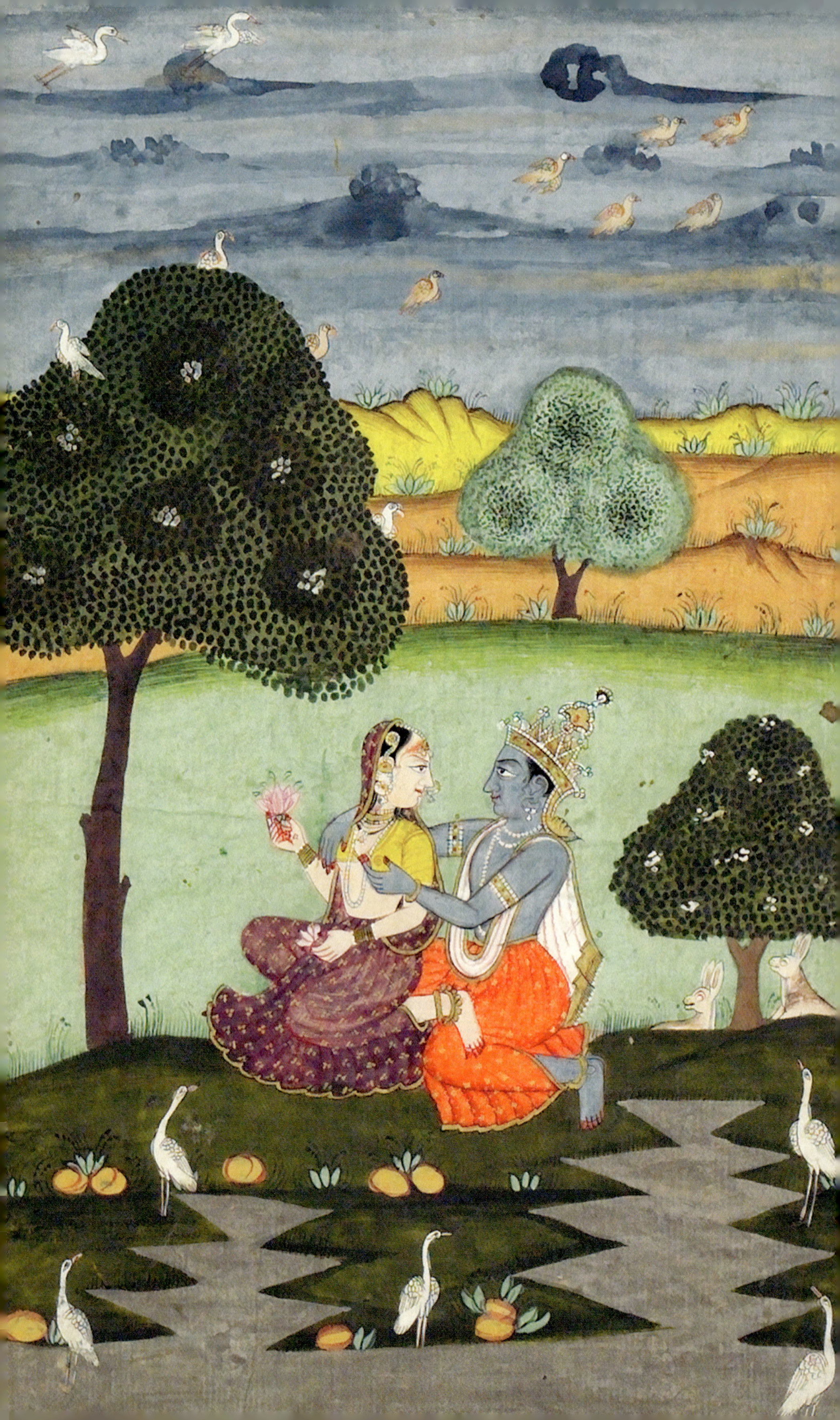

Part One: Introductory Preface

Chapter I Salutation to virtue, wealth and pleasure

Sutras 1–4 Salutation to Dharma, Artha and Kama, the Three Aims of Life that are dealt with in this *shastra* [treatise].[1] Salutation also to those masters who have made a thorough study of these subjects, and to those sages who have spread their teaching. The work of both has great bearing on the present subject.

Sutras 5–10 In the beginning, the Lord of Beings created men and women, and in 100,000 chapters laid down rules for regulating their existence with regard to Dharma, Artha and Kama. Some of these, namely those which dealt with Dharma, were separately written by Swayambhu Manu; those that related to Artha were compiled by Brihaspati; and those that referred to Kama were expounded by Nandi, the follower of Mahadeva, in 1,000 chapters.

Then these "Kama Sutra" (Aphorisms on Love), written by Nandi in 1,000 chapters, were reproduced by Shvetaketu, the son of Uddvalaka, in an abbreviated form in 500 chapters, which was in turn abridged, in 150 chapters, by Babhravya, of the Panchala region. These 150 chapters were then arranged into seven parts named: *Sadharana* (general topics), *Samprayogika* (embraces, and so on), *Kanya Samprayuktaka* (union of males and females), *Bharyadhikarika* (on one's own wife), *Paradika* (on the wives of other men), *Vaisika* (on courtesans) and *Aupamishadika* (on the arts of seduction, tonic medicines,[2] and so on).

Sutras 11–17 The sixth part was separately expounded by Dattaka at the request of the "public women" [courtesans; see note 16] of

Pataliputra (Patna), and following this example Charayana explained the first part. The remaining parts – the second, third, fourth, fifth and seventh – were each separately expounded by Suvarnanabha, Ghotakamukha, Gonardiya, Gonikaputra and Kuchumara, respectively.

Thus the work, being written in parts by different authors, became almost unobtainable, and because the original work of Babhravya was difficult to master on account of its length, and the parts which were expounded by Dattaka and the others dealt only with particular branches of the subject, Vatsyayana therefore composed his work in a small volume as an abstract of the works of the above named authors.

Chapter II On the acquisition of virtue, wealth and pleasure

Sutra 1 Man, the period of whose life is 100 years, should practise Dharma, Artha and Kama at different times and in such a manner that they may harmonize and not clash in any way.

Sutras 2–4 He should acquire learning in his childhood, in his youth and middle age he should attend to Artha and Kama, and in his old age he should perform Dharma, and thus seek to gain *moksha.*[3]

Sutras 5–6 Or, on account of the uncertainty of life, he may practise them at times of his choosing. But he should lead the life of a religious student until he has finished his education.

Sutras 7–8 Dharma is obedience to the command of the *shastra* or acting in accordance with the *sruti*,[4] such as by the performance of sacrifices, which are not generally done, because they do not belong to this world, and produce no visible effect; and not to do other things, such as eating meat, which is often done because it belongs to this world, and has visible effects. Dharma should be learned from the *sruti*, and from those conversant with them.

Sutras 9–10 Artha is the acquisition of arts, land, gold, cattle, wealth, equipment and friends. It is, further, the protection of what is acquired, and the increase of what is protected.

Artha should be learned from the king's officers, and from merchants who may be versed in the ways of commerce.

Sutras 11–13 Kama is the enjoyment of appropriate objects by the five senses of hearing, touch, sight, taste and smell, assisted by the mind and the soul. Kama is actually a peculiar contact between the organ of sense and its object – one which gives rise to the consciousness of pleasure.

Kama is to be learned from the *Kama Sutra* and from worldly citizens.

Sutras 14–17 When all three – Dharma, Artha and Kama – come together, the former is better than the one which follows it. That is, Dharma is better than Artha, and Artha is better than Kama. But Artha should always be the first to be practised by the king, for the livelihood of men is to be obtained from it only. Again, Kama being the occupation of courtesans, they should prefer it to the other two, and these are exceptions to the general rule.

Objection 1

Sutras 18–21 Some learned men say that because Dharma is connected with things not belonging to this world, it is appropriate to discuss it in a book; similarly, Artha is practised by the application of certain methods and a knowledge of those can only be obtained by study and from books. But Kama being a thing that is practised even by the animal world, and which is to be found everywhere, does not require any learned work on the subject.

Answer

Sutras 22–24 This is not so. Sexual intercourse being a thing dependent on man and woman necessitates the use of proper actions and those actions are to be learned from the *Kama Sutra*. Proper actions are absent in the animal world, caused by animals being unrestrained and by the females among them being fit for sexual intercourse only at certain seasons and no more, and by their intercourse not being preceded by thought of any kind.

Objection 2

Sutras 25–30 The Lokayatikas[5] say that religious ordinances should not be observed, because they bear fruit only in the future, and indeed it is doubtful whether they will bear any fruit at all. What foolish person will give away that which is in his own hands into the hands of another? Moreover, it is better to have a pigeon today than a peacock tomorrow; and a copper coin that we have the certainty of obtaining is better than a gold coin, the possession of which is doubtful.

Answer

Sutra 31 It is not so.

First, the *sruti* which ordain the practice of Dharma do not admit of a doubt.

Second, sacrifices such as those made for the destruction of enemies, or for the fall of rain, are seen to bear fruit.

Third, the sun, moon, stars, planets and other heavenly bodies appear to work intentionally for the good of the world.

Fourth, the existence of this world is affected by the observance of the rules respecting the four classes of men and their four stages of life.[6]

Fifth, we see that seed is sown in anticipation of future crops.

Vatsyayana is therefore of the opinion that the ordinances of religion must be obeyed.

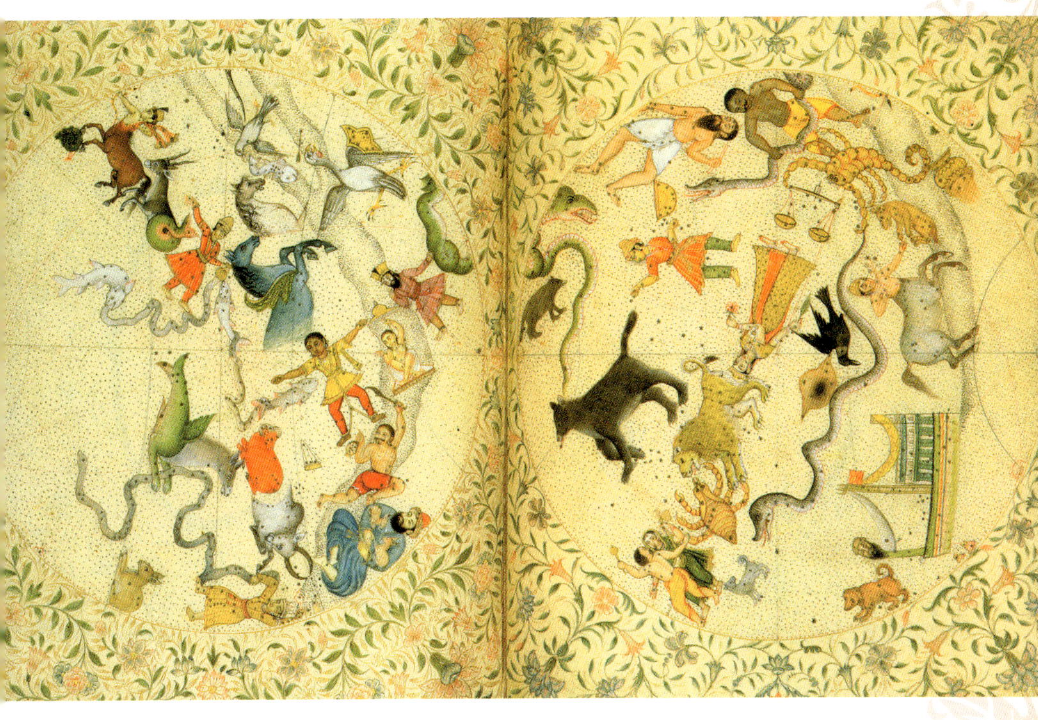

Objection 3

Sutras 32–37 Those who believe that destiny is the prime mover of all things say that we should not strive to acquire wealth, for sometimes it is not acquired despite our effort, while at other times it comes to us of itself without any exertion on our part. Everything is therefore in the power of destiny, who is the lord of gain and loss, of success and defeat, of pleasure and pain. Thus we see that it was destiny that raised Bali[7] to the throne of Indra, it was the same power that caused his downfall, and it is only destiny that can reinstate him.

Answer

Sutras 38–39 It is not right to say so. Because the acquisition of every object presupposes some exertion on the part of man, the application of proper means may be said to be the cause of gaining all our ends, and this application of proper means being thus necessary (even where a thing is destined to happen), it follows that a person who does nothing will enjoy no happiness.

Objection 4

Sutras 40–45 Those who are inclined to think that Artha is the chief object to be obtained argue thus. Pleasures should not be sought for; they are obstacles to the practice of Dharma and Artha, which are both superior to them, and are also disliked by meritorious persons. Pleasures also bring a man into distress, and into contact with low persons; they cause him to commit unrighteous deeds, and produce impurity in him; they make him regardless of the future, and encourage carelessness and levity. And lastly, they cause him to be disbelieved by all, received by none, and despised by everybody, including himself. It is notorious, moreover, that many men who have given themselves up solely to pleasure have been ruined along with their families and relations. Thus, King Dandakya, of the Bhoja dynasty, carried off a Brahmin's daughter with evil intent, and was eventually ruined and lost his kingdom. Indra, too, having violated the chastity of Ahalya, was made to suffer for it. In a like manner the mighty Kichaka, who tried to seduce Draupadi, and Ravana, who attempted to win over Sita, were punished for their crimes. These and many others fell by reason of their subjection to Kama.

Answer

Sutras 46–48 This objection cannot be sustained, for pleasures are as necessary for the existence and well-being of the body as is food, and consequently equally required. They are, moreover, the results of Dharma and Artha. Therefore, pleasures are to be followed with moderation and caution. No one refrains from cooking food because there are beggars asking for it, or from sowing seed because there are deer that will destroy the corn as it grows.

Sutras 49–51 In this way a man practising Dharma, Artha and Kama enjoys happiness both in this world and in the world to come. The wise perform those actions in which there is no fear as to what is to result from them in the next world, and in which there is no danger to their welfare. Any action which is conducive to the practice of Dharma, Artha and Kama together, or of any two, or even one of them, should be performed, but an action which is conducive to the practice of one of them at the expense of the remaining two should not be performed.

Chapter III On the arts and sciences to be studied

Sutras 1–4 Man should study the *Kama Sutra* and its subsidiary arts and sciences alongside the study of the arts and sciences in Dharma and Artha. Even young maids should study this *Kama Sutra* along with its arts and sciences before marriage, and after it they should continue to do so with the consent of their husbands.

Here some learned men object, and say that females, not being allowed to study any science, should not study the *Kama Sutra*.

Sutras 5–11 But Vatsyayana contends that this objection does not hold good, for women already know the practice of *Kama Sutra*, and that practice is derived from the *Kama Shastra*, or the science of Kama itself. Moreover, there are many cases where the practice of a science is known to all, but only a few persons are acquainted with the rules and laws on which it is based. Thus the *yadnika*s or sacrificers, though ignorant of grammar, make use of appropriate words when addressing the different deities, and do not know how these words are framed. Again, persons do the duties required of them on auspicious days, which are fixed by astrology, though they are not acquainted with the science of astrology. In a like manner riders of horses and elephants train these animals without knowing the science of training animals, but from practice only. And similarly the people of the most distant provinces obey the laws of the kingdom from customary practice, and because there is a king over them, and without further reason.

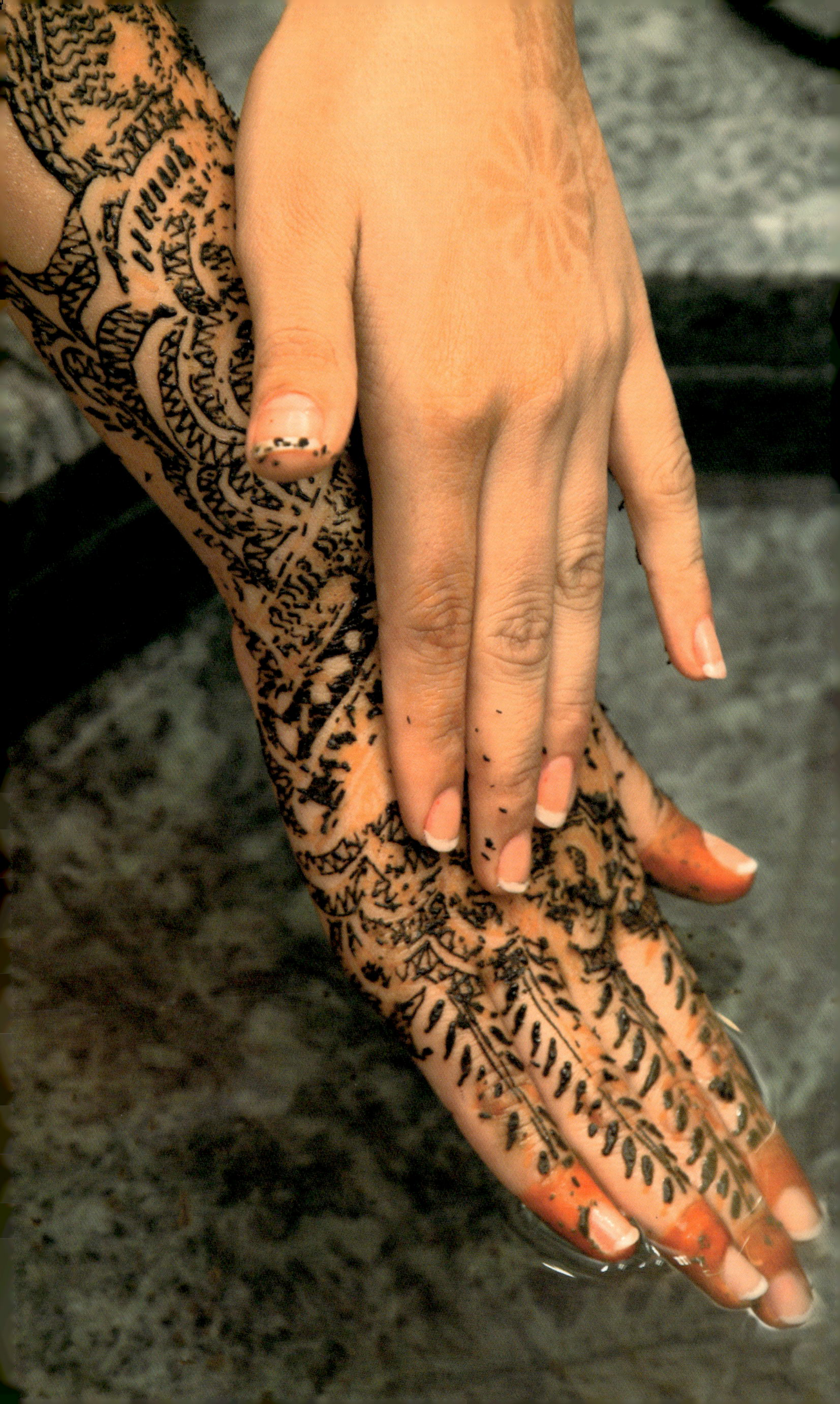

Sutra 12 And from experience we find that some women, such as princesses, the daughters of ministers and courtesans, are actually versed in the *Kama Shastra*.

Sutra 13 A female, therefore, should learn the *Kama Shastra*, or at least a part of it, by studying it with the help of a confidante.

Sutra 14 She should study alone in private the sixty-four practices that form a part of the *Kama Shastra*.

Sutra 15 Her teacher should be [married and] one of the following: the daughter of a nurse brought up with her, a female friend who can be trusted in everything, a cousin and an equal in age, an old female servant, a female beggar who may once have lived in the family, or her own sister who can always be trusted.

Sutras 16–19 The following are the sixty-four arts to be studied, together with the *Kama Sutra*:

Singing
Playing musical instruments
Dancing
Dancing, singing, and playing musical instruments
Writing and drawing
Tattooing
Arraying and adorning an idol with rice and flowers
Spreading and arranging beds, settees or divans
Colouring teeth, garments, hair, nails and bodies
Fixing stained glass into a floor
The art of making beds, and spreading out carpets and cushions for reclining
Creating music with water

Collecting and storing water in aqueducts, cisterns and reservoirs
Picture making, trimming and decorating
Stringing of rosaries, necklaces, garlands and wreaths
Binding of turbans and making head decorations of flowers
Scenic representations
Art of making ear ornaments
Art of preparing perfumes and odours
Proper arrangement of jewels, decorations, and adornment in dress
Magic or creating illusion
Quickness of hand or deft manual skill
Cooking and culinary arts
Making lemonades, sherbets and drinks with flavour and colour
Needlework
Making patterns (parrot motif, flower motif, tassels, and so on)
Solving of riddles, enigmas, verbal puzzles and enigmatic questions
A game in which one party recites a verse and the other party has to respond immediately with a verse that begins with the same letter with which the last speaker's verse ended
The arts of mimicry, imitation and impersonation
Reading, including chanting and intoning
Study of sentences that are difficult to pronounce correctly when repeated quickly
Practice with sword, single stick, quarter staff and bow and arrow
Drawing inferences, reasoning or inferring
Carpentry, or making furniture for sitting and reclining
Knowledge of the art of building
Distinguishing between precious and non-precious metals and jewels
Chemistry and the study of minerals
Colouring jewels, gems and beads
Knowledge of mines and quarries
Gardening and horticulture, including a knowledge of how to treat

disease among trees and plants, how to nourish them and how to determine age

Art of cock-fighting, quail-fighting and ram-fighting

Art of teaching parrots and myna birds to speak

Art of applying perfumed ointments to the body, and of dressing the hair with unguents and perfumes and braiding it

The art of understanding writing in cipher, and the writing of words in a peculiar way

The art of speaking by changing the word forms of words: by altering the beginning and end of words, by adding unnecessary letters between every syllable of a word, and so on

Knowledge of other regional languages and dialects

Art of making flower carriages

Art of addressing spells and charms, and binding armlets

Mental exercises, such as completing stanzas or verses on receiving a part of them; or supplying one, two or three lines when the remaining lines are given indiscriminately from different verses, so as to make a whole verse with meaning; or arranging the words of a verse written irregularly by separating the vowels from the consonants, or leaving them out altogether. There are many other such exercises.

Composing poems

Knowledge of dictionaries and vocabularies

Knowledge of ways of disguising the appearance of persons

Knowledge of the art of changing the appearance of things, such as making cotton to appear as silk, coarse and common things to appear as fine and good

Various ways of gambling

Art of obtaining possession of the property of others by means of incantations

Skill in youthful sports

Knowledge of social etiquette
Knowledge of the art of war, of arms, of armies, and so on
Knowledge of gymnastics
Art of knowing the character of a man from his features
Knowledge of scanning or constructing verses
Arithmetical games
Making artificial flowers
Making figures and images in clay

Sutra 20 A courtesan, endowed with a good disposition, beauty and other winning qualities, who is also versed in the above arts, obtains the rank of Ganika, or courtesan of high quality, and receives a seat of honour in a gathering of men.

Sutra 21 Such a woman is respected by the king and praised by learned men, and since she is sought after by all she enjoys universal regard.

Sutra 22 A princess or the daughter of a minister, being learned in the above arts, can make their husbands favourable to them, even though these may have thousands of other wives besides themselves.

Sutra 23 And in the same manner, if a wife becomes separated from her husband, and falls into distress, she can support herself easily, even in a foreign country, by means of her knowledge of these arts. Even the bare knowledge of them gives attractiveness to a woman, though the practice of them may be only possible or otherwise according to the circumstances of each case.

Sutra 24 A man who is versed in these arts, who is loquacious and acquainted with the arts of gallantry, soon gains the hearts of women, even though he is only known to them for a short time.

Chapter IV The life of a citizen

Sutra 1 Having acquired learning, a man, with the wealth that he may have gained by gift, conquest, purchase, deposit,[8] or inheritance from his ancestors, should assume the life and duties of a cultivated citizen.

Sutras 2–3 He should take a house in a city, or large village, or in the vicinity of cultivated and refined people, or in a place which is the resort of such persons.

Sutra 4 This house should be situated near some water, and divided into different compartments for different domestic purposes. It should be surrounded by a garden, and also contain two rooms, an outer and an inner one.

Sutra 5 The inner room should be occupied by the females, while the outer room, made balmy with rich perfumes, should contain a soft, low

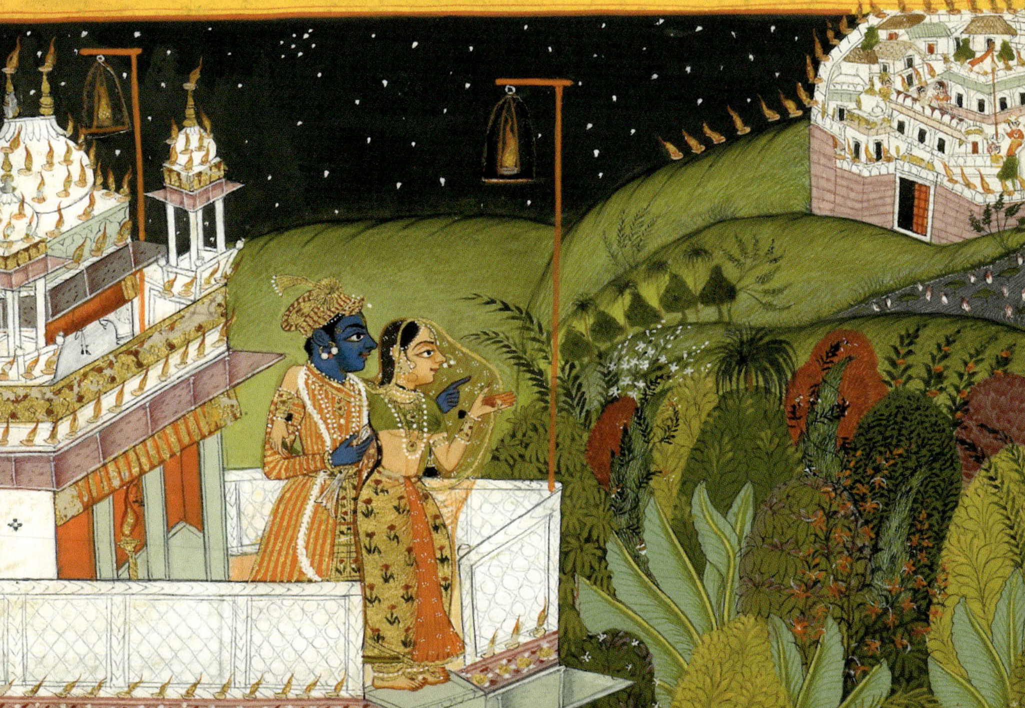

bed covered with clean white bedlinen, with garlands and bunches of natural garden flowers upon it, a canopy above it, and two pillows, one at the top and another at the bottom. There should also be a sort of couch nearby.

Sutras 6–8 At the head of this couch, a sort of stool, there should be placed fragrant ointments for the night, as well as flowers, pots containing collyrium and other fragrant substances, things used to perfume the mouth, and the bark of the common citron tree.

Sutra 9 Near the couch, on the ground, there should be a spittoon.

Sutra 10 There should be a box containing ornaments, and also a *veena* [lute-like stringed instrument] hanging from an ivory peg, a board for drawing, a pot containing perfume, some books, and some garlands of the yellow amaranth flowers.

Sutra 11 Not far from the couch, on the ground, there should be a round mat with a cushion.

Sutra 12 Also nearby should be a toy cart and a board for playing games with dice.

Sutra 13 Outside the outer room there should be cages of birds such as quails, partridges, parrots, mynas, and so on.

Sutra 14 Usually there is a separate place for the making of artificial aids for sexual congress.

Sutra 15 In the garden there should be a whirling swing and a common swing, set within a shady canopy of creepers covered with flowers.

Sutra 16 The citizen, having got up and performed any calls of nature, should wash his teeth, apply some ointments and perfumes to his body, put some ornaments on his person and collyrium[9] on his eyelids and below his eyes, colour his lips with *alacktaka*,[10] and view himself in the looking glass. Having then eaten betel leaves and given a sweet-smelling fragrance to the mouth, he should go about his usual business.

Sutra 17 He should bathe daily, anoint his limbs with oil every other day, apply a lathering substance[11] to his body every three days, get his head (including face) shaved every four days and all the other parts of his body every five or ten days.[12]

Sutra 18 All these things should be done without fail, and the sweat of the armpits should also be removed.

Sutras 19–20 Meals should be taken at breakfast and in the afternoon. Charayana (see page 18) is of the same opinion in this matter.

Sutra 21 After breakfast, parrots and mynas should be taught to speak, and fights involving cocks, quails and rams should be watched. A limited time should be devoted to entertaining diversions with the *pithamarda*, the *vita* and the *vidushaka*,[13] followed by a midday siesta.[14]

Sutra 22 After that the citizen, having put on his clothes, should converse with his friends during the afternoon.

Sutra 23 In the evening there should be singing.

Sutra 24 After that the citizen and his friends should await the ladies' arrival in his room, which will have been decorated and perfumed. He may send a female messenger for them, or fetch them himself.

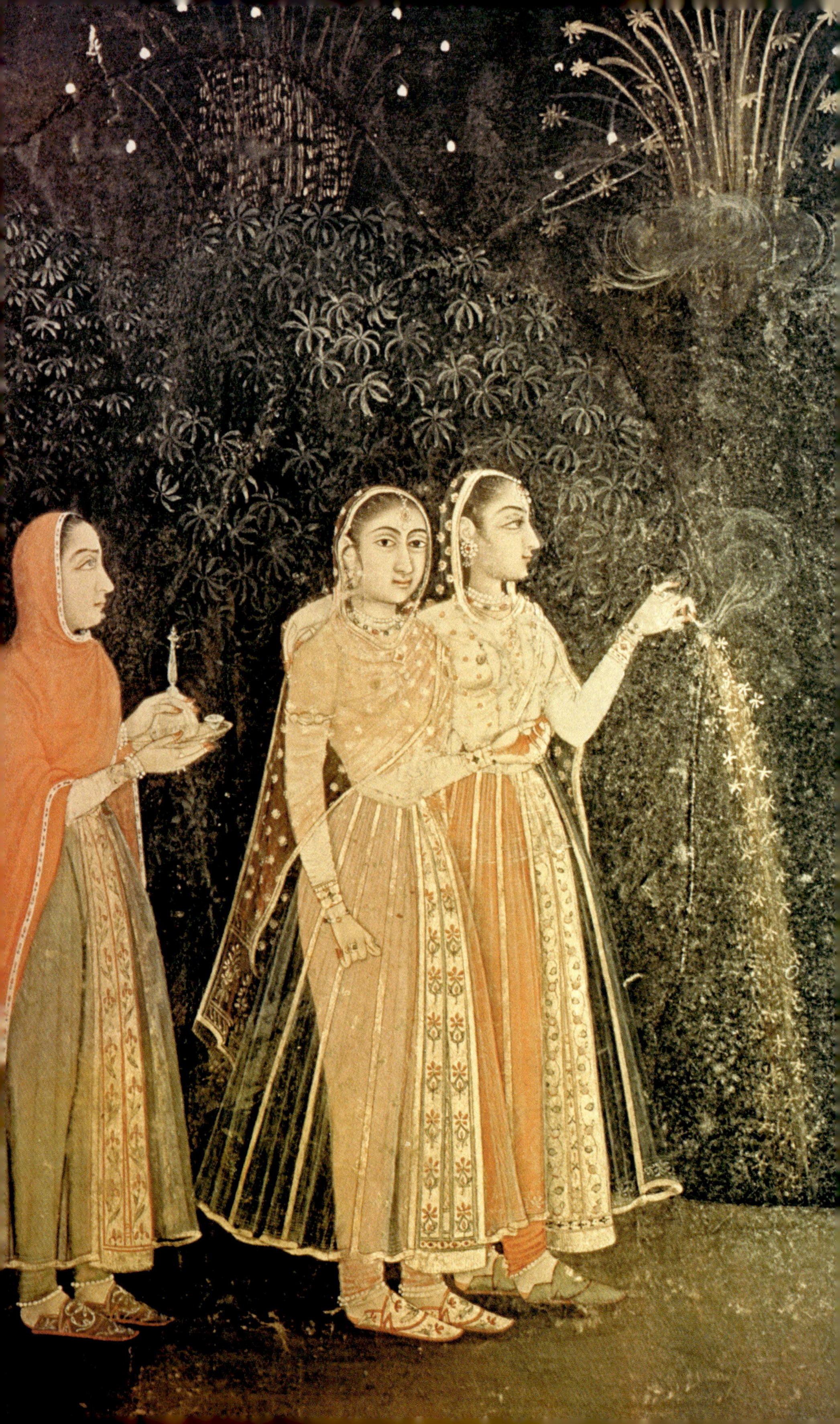

Sutra 25 After their arrival at his house, he and his friends should welcome them and entertain them with loving and agreeable conversation. Thus end the duties of the day.

Sutra 26 The following things are to be undertaken occasionally as diversions or amusements: holding festivals in honour of different deities; social gatherings of both sexes; drinking parties; picnics; and sports and other social diversions.

Festivals

Sutras 27–33 On particular auspicious days an assembly of citizens should be convened in the temple of Saraswati.[15] There the skill of singers, and of others who may have come recently to the town, should be tested, and on the following day they should always be given some rewards. After that the singers may either be retained or dismissed, according to how their performances were liked or not by the assembly. The members of the assembly should act in concert, both in times of distress as well as in times of prosperity, and it is also the duty of these citizens to show hospitality to strangers who may have come to the assembly from afar. What is said above should be understood to apply to all the other festivals which may be held in honour of the different deities, according to the present rules.

Social gatherings

Sutras 34–36 When men of the same age, disposition and talents, who are fond of the same diversions and possess the same degree of education, sit together at the house of one of them or of a courtesan,[16] or in an assembly of citizens, to engage in agreeable discourse with each other, it is called a "sitting in company" or a social gathering. Discussions include the completion of verses half composed by others and testing the knowledge of one another in the various arts. The women, who may be the most beautiful, who may like the same things that the men like, and who may have power to attract the minds of others, are shown special respect.

Drinking parties

Sutras 37–38 Men and women should take turns to drink in one another's houses. And here there should be drunk liquors which are of bitter and sour taste; also drinks concocted from the barks of various trees, wild fruits and leaves.

Picnics

Sutras 39–40 In the forenoon, having dressed themselves men should make an excursion on horseback, accompanied by courtesans and followed by servants. And having performed the day's duties and passed the time with various agreeable diversions, such as the fighting of quails, cocks and rams, and other spectacles, they should return home in the afternoon in the same manner, bringing with them mementos, such as bunches of flowers, and so on.

Sports and other social diversions

Sutras 41–42 When bathing in summer any dangerous animals should have been removed from these watery places, which should also have been built in on all sides.

Nights can be spent playing with dice.

Moonlight nights can be celebrated with swinging, and so on.

Other special games include:

Maintaining the festive day in honour of spring.

Plucking the sprouts and fruits of the mango trees.

Eating the stalks of lotuses.

Eating the tender ears of corn.

Picnicking in the forests when the trees get their new foliage.

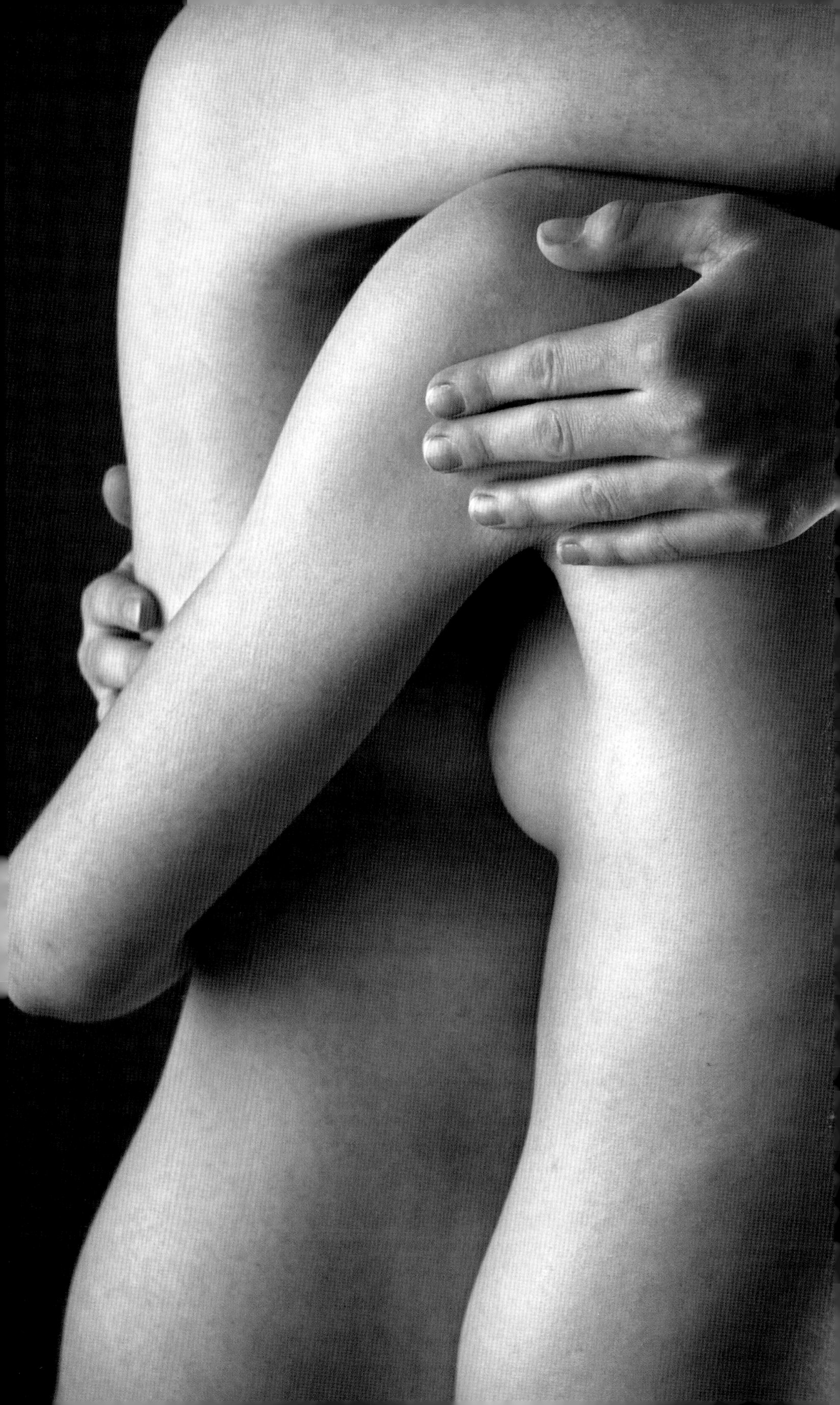

The Udakakashvedika or sporting play with water.

Decorating each other with the flowers of some trees.

Pelting each other with the flowers of the kadamba tree, and many other sports which may be known only in some parts of the country.

Citizens should always carry on these and similar other amusements.

Sutra 43 The above amusements should be followed by a person who diverts himself on his own in company with a courtesan, as well as by a courtesan who can do the same with her maidservants or with citizens.

Sutras 44–47 A *pithamarda*[17] is a man without wealth whose only property consists of his *mallika*,[18] some lathering substance and a red cloth, who comes from a good part of the country, and who is well versed in the arts; and by practising these arts he makes a living and is received in the company of citizens and in the home of courtesans.

A *vita*[19] is a man who has enjoyed good fortune and tasted life's pleasures, is a compatriot of the citizens with whom he associates, has the good qualities of a citizen, has a wife, and is honoured in the assembly of citizens and in the homes of courtesans, and depends on them for his livelihood.

A *vidushaka*[20] (also called a *vaihasaka*, that is, one who provokes laughter) is a person acquainted with only some of the arts, who is mainly a jester, and trusted by all.

These persons are employed to mediate between citizens and public women and reconcile them after quarrels.

Sutra 48 This remark applies also to female mendicants, to women with their heads shaved, to adulterous women, and to aged courtesans.

Sutra 49 Thus a citizen respected by all in his town or village should call on those of his own caste who may be worth knowing. He should converse in company and gratify his friends by his sociability, and by assisting them with various matters he should cause them to assist one another in the same way.

Sutra 50 A citizen conversing not entirely in Sanskrit,[21] nor wholly in a regional dialect, will obtain great respect.

Sutra 51 The wise should avoid gatherings disliked by the public, not governed by any rules, and intent on maligning others.

Sutra 52 A wise man who attends gatherings approved of by the public, at which the only object is pleasure, will be highly respected.

Chapter V About the kinds of women to consort with, and friends and messengers

Sutras 1–3 When Kama is practised by men of the four castes according to the rules of the Holy Writ (that is, by lawful marriage) with virgins of their own caste, it becomes a means of acquiring lawful progeny and good fame, and it is not against custom. However, the practice of Kama with women of the higher castes, and with those previously enjoyed by others, even though they be of the same caste, is prohibited. The practice of Kama with women of the lower castes, with women excommunicated from their caste, with courtesans, and with women "twice married",[22] is neither urged nor condemned. The object of practising Kama with such women is pleasure only.

Sutra 4 Therefore *nayikas*[23] are of three kinds: the maiden, the woman "twice married" and the courtesan.

Sutra 5 According to Gonikaputra there is a fourth kind of *nayika*: one who is married to another but who is resorted to on some special occasion (other than for procreation or pleasure).

Sutras 6–7 These special occasions are when a man thinks in this way: This woman is self-willed, and has been previously enjoyed by many others besides me. I may, therefore, safely resort to her like a courtesan, though she belongs to a higher caste than mine, and, in so doing, I shall not be violating the ordinances of Dharma.

Or in this way: This is a "twice-married woman" and she has been enjoyed by others before me; there is, therefore, no objection to my resorting to her.

Sutra 8 Or in this way: This woman has gained the heart of her great and powerful husband, and exercises a mastery over him, who is a friend of my enemy; if, therefore, she becomes united with me she will cause her husband to abandon my enemy.

Sutra 9 Or in this way: This woman will turn the mind of her husband, who is very powerful, in my favour, he being at present disaffected toward me and intent on doing me some harm.

Sutra 10 Or in this way: By making this woman my friend I shall gain the object of some friend of mine, or shall be able to effect the ruin of some enemy, or shall accomplish some other difficult purpose.

Sutra 11 Or in this way: By being united with this woman, I shall kill her husband and so obtain his vast riches, which I covet.

Sutra 12 Or in this way: The union of this woman with me is not dangerous, and because I am poor it will bring me the wealth I need. I shall therefore obtain her vast riches in this way without any difficulty.

Sutra 13–15 Or in this way: This woman loves me ardently, and she knows all my weak points; if, therefore, I am unwilling to be with her, she will make my faults public and thus tarnish my reputation. Or she will bring some gross accusation against me, of which it may be hard to clear myself and I shall be ruined. Or perhaps she will detach from me her husband who is powerful, and yet under her control, and she will unite him with my enemy, or she will herself join my enemy.

Sutra 16 Or in this way: The husband of this woman has violated my wives. I shall therefore pay him back by seducing his wives.

Sutra 17 Or in this way: By the help of this woman I shall kill an enemy of the king, who has taken shelter with her, and whom I am ordered by the king to destroy.

Sutra 18 Or in this way: The woman whom I love is under the control of this woman. I shall, through the influence of the latter, be able to get at the former.

Sutra 19 Or in this way: This woman will bring to me a maid, who possesses wealth and beauty, but who is hard to get at, and under the control of another.

Sutra 20–21 Or lastly in this way: My enemy is a friend of this woman's husband. I shall therefore cause her to join him, and will thus create an enmity between her husband and him.

For these and other similar motives, the wives of other men may be resorted to, but it must be understood clearly that it is allowed only for special reasons and not for mere carnal desire.

Sutra 22 Charayana thinks that under these circumstances there is also

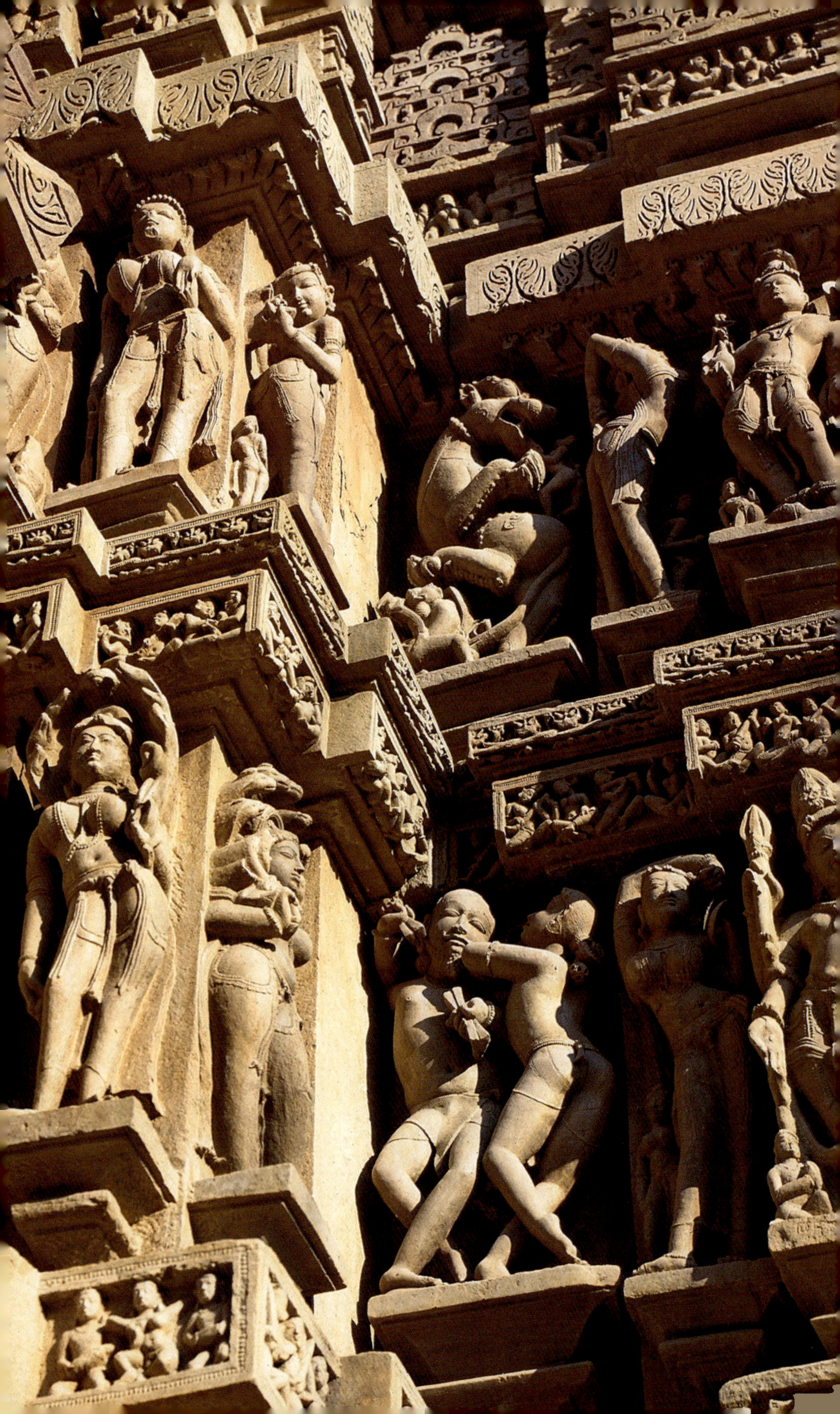

a fifth kind of *nayika*: a woman who is kept by a minister, or who repairs to him occasionally; or a widow who accomplishes the purpose of a man with the person to whom she resorts.

Sutra 23 Suvarnanabha adds that a widow who has renounced the world may be considered as a sixth kind of *nayika*.

Sutra 24 Ghotakamukha says that a seventh kind of *nayika* is formed by the unmarried daughters of courtesans or maidservants.

Sutra 25 Gonardiya puts forth his doctrine that any woman born of good family, after she has come of age, is an eighth kind of *nayika*.

Sutras 26–27 But these latter four kinds of *nayika*s do not differ much from the first four kinds, because the motives for resorting to them are the same. Therefore, Vatsyayana is of the opinion that there are only four kinds of *nayika*s: the maiden, the woman "twice married", the courtesan and the woman resorted to for a special purpose.

Sutras 28–31 There is one type of *nayaka* for all *nayika*s, one who accomplishes things in complete secrecy. This class of *nayaka* divides into three groups: the best, the better and the lowest type, depending on his qualifications. The qualifications of both *nayaka*s and *nayika*s will be described when dealing with courtesans. [See pages 200–245.]

Sutra 32 Physical union with the following types of woman is forbidden: a leper, a lunatic, a woman turned out of caste, a woman who reveals secrets, a woman who publicly expresses desire for sexual intercourse, a woman who is extremely white, a woman who is extremely black, a bad-smelling woman, a woman who is a near relation, a woman who is a female friend, a woman who leads the life of an ascetic or recluse, and, lastly, the wife of a relation, the wife of a friend, the wife of a learned Brahmin or the wife of a ruler.

Sutra 33 The followers of Babhravya say that any woman who has relations with five men is a fit and proper person to resort to.

Sutra 34 But Gonikaputra urges that even when this is the case, the wives of relations, learned Brahmins and kings are excepted.

Sutra 35 The following describes kinds of friends: one who has played with you in childhood; one who is bound by an obligation; one who is of the same disposition and fond of the same things; one who is a fellow student; one who is acquainted with your secrets and faults, and whose faults and secrets are known to you; one who is a child of your nurse; one who is brought up with you; and one who is a hereditary friend.

Sutra 36 These friends should possess the following qualities: they should tell the truth; they should not be changed by time; they should be favourable to your designs; they should be firm in friendship; they should be free from covetousness; they should be dependable; and they should not reveal your secrets.

Sutras 37–38 Charayana says that friends of the citizen may include washermen, barbers, cowherds, florists, druggists, betel-leaf sellers, tavern-keepers, beggars, *pithamarda*s, *vita*s and *vidushaka*s, and the wives of all these people.

Sutra 39 Any person who is a friend of both the citizen and the *nayika*, loving them equally but more trusted by the *nayika*, can perform the function of a love messenger.

Sutra 40 A messenger should possess the following qualities: skilfulness, boldness, an ability to read others' intentions, forthrightness, an insight into others' behaviour and motives, good manners, an awareness of the propriety of time and place, business ingenuity, quickness of comprehension, and resourcefulness.

Sutra 41 And this part ends with a verse: "The man who is ingenious and wise, who is accompanied by a friend, and who knows the intentions of others, and the proper time and place for doing everything, can win over even a woman who is hard to be obtained."

NOTES

1. The Three Aims of Life are Dharma, Artha and Kama: Dharma is the acquisition of religious merit, or virtue, as well as ethical conduct and rules pertaining to social class; Artha is the acquisition of material wealth; and Kama is pleasure and sensual gratification.
2. "Medicines" here refer to love-making aids.
3. Release from the cycle of death and rebirth.
4. Hindu sacred texts.
5. Followers of an essentially materialist system.
6. The four classes of Hindu men are the Brahmin, or priestly class; the Kshatriya, or warrior class; the Vaishya, or mercantile class; and the Shudra, or menial class. The four stages of life are: religious student, householder, hermit and devotee.
7. Bali was a demon who had conquered Indra and gained his throne, but was later overcome by Vishnu at the time of his fifth incarnation.
8. Gift is peculiar to a Brahmin, conquest to a Kshatraya, while purchase, deposit and other means of acquiring wealth belong to the Vaishya.
9. Collyrium is an eye salve in dry or liquid form.
10. *Alacktaka* was made using lac, a scarlet pigment secreted by certain insects.
11. Used instead of soap.
12. Hairs are plucked after ten days.
13. *Pithamarda*, *vita* and *vidushaka* are stock character-types in ancient Indian drama. See *sutras* 44–47 [page 36] and related Notes.
14. Midday sleep is only allowed in summer.
15. Deity adored as the patroness of the fine arts, especially of music and rhetoric, the inventor of Sanskrit and goddess of harmony and eloquence.
16. The "public women", or courtesans (*vesya*), of the ancient Hindus have often been compared with the *hetaera* of the Greeks.
17. A sort of professor of all the arts, who as such is received as the friend and confidante of the citizens.
18. A seat in the form of the letter T
19. Like the character of the parasite in Greek comedy, perhaps retained by the wealthy and dissipated as a private instructor as well as an entertaining companion.
20. Evidently the buffoon or jester. Always a Brahmin, a man of rank, who is shrewd yet simple, fond of good living and with a love of ease. He is to excite mirth by being ridiculous.
21. It is presumed that this means the citizen should be acquainted with several languages. The middle part of this paragraph might apply to secret societies – it was perhaps a reference to the Thugs.
22. Not a widow but a woman who has probably left her husband and is living with someone as a married woman.
23. *Nayika* refers to a female beloved, *nayaka* to a male lover. A *nayika* is any woman fit to be enjoyed without sin for the purpose of pleasure or progeny. However, there is another kind of *nayika* admitted to later, enjoyed neither for pleasure nor for progeny, but merely for accomplishing a purpose.

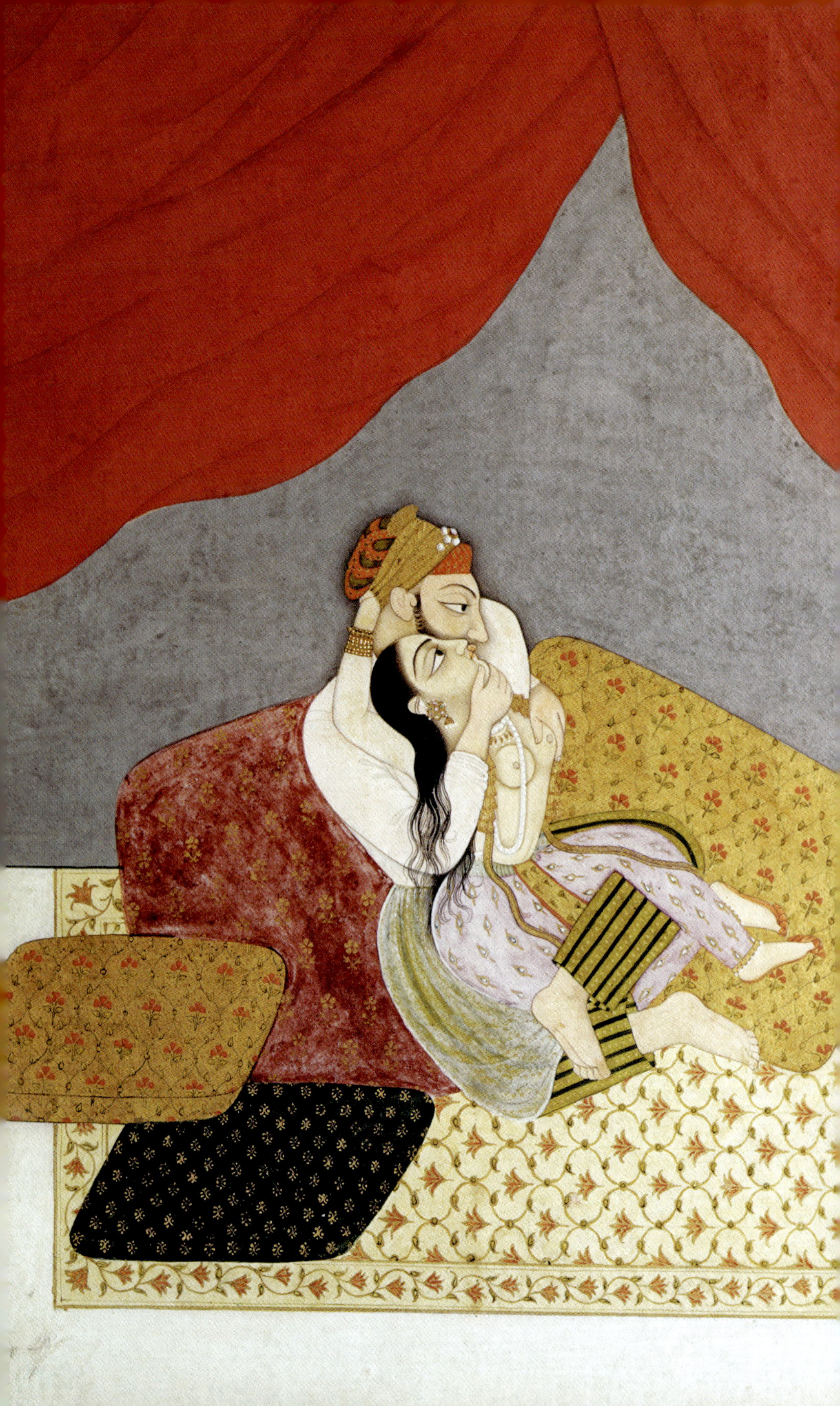

Part Two: On Sexual Union

Chapter I Kinds of sexual union according to dimension, intensity of passion and duration

Kinds of union

Sutra 1 Men can be divided into three types according to the size of their *lingam*[1] – the hare type (small), the bull type (medium) and the horse type (large).

Sutra 2 Women can be divided into three types according to the depth of their *yoni*[2] – the deer type (small), the mare type (medium) and the elephant type (large).

Sutras 3–4 There are thus three equal unions between persons of corresponding dimensions, and there are six unequal unions, when the dimensions do not correspond, making a total of nine unions in all:

Equal: Hare and deer, bull and mare, horse and elephant.

Unequal: Hare and mare, hare and elephant, bull and deer, bull and elephant, horse and deer, horse and mare.

Sutras 5–6 In these unequal unions, when the male exceeds the female in dimension, his union with a woman immediately next to him in size is called a high union, and is of two kinds, while his union with a woman most remote from him in size is called the highest union, and is of one kind only.

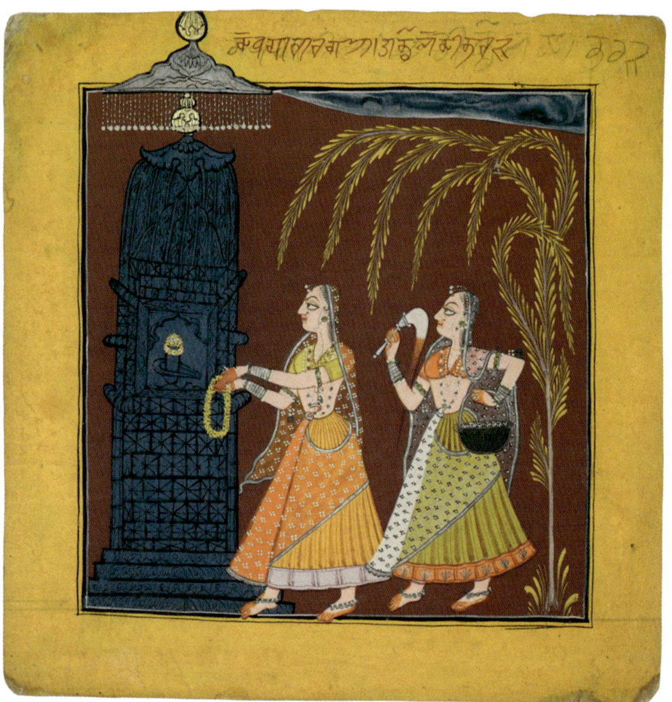

Sutras 7–8 On the other hand, when the female exceeds the male in size, her union with a man immediately next to her in size is called a low union, and is of two kinds, while her union with a man most distant from her in size is called the lowest union, and is of one kind only.

Sutras 9–12 In other words, the horse and mare, the bull and deer, form a high union, while the horse and deer form the highest union. On the female side, the elephant and bull, the mare and hare, form a low union, while the elephant and hare form the lowest union. There are, then, nine kinds of union according to dimensions. Equal unions are the best; those of a superlative degree, that is the highest and the lowest, are the worst; and the rest are middling, and with them the high ones are better than the low ones.[3]

There are also nine kinds of union according to the intensity of passion or desire, as follows:

Equal: small and small, middling and middling, intense and intense.

Unequal: small and middling, small and intense, middling and small, middling and intense, intense and small, intense and middling.

Sutras 13–14 A man is one of small passion when his desire at the time of sexual union is not great, who cannot bear the warm embraces of the female and whose semen is meagre. A man with greater desire is of middling passion, while one full of desire has intense passion.

Sutras 15–16 In the same way, women are supposed to have the three degrees of feeling, and nine different combinations, as specified above.

Sutra 17 Lastly, according to duration there are three kinds of men and women: the short-timed, the moderate-timed and the long-timed; and of these, as in the previous statements, there are nine kinds of union.

Sutra 18 But on the subject of duration there is a difference of opinion about the female, which should be stated.

Sutras 19–25 Auddalika says: "Females do not exhibit pleasure through emission as males do. The female takes a kind of pleasure from the consciousness of desire, which gives her a satisfaction totally different from the male, but it is impossible for them to tell you what kind of pleasure they feel. The fact from which this becomes evident is that males, when engaged in coition, cease of themselves after emission and are satisfied, but it is not so with females."

Sutra 26 This opinion is disputed on the grounds that females love men who perform more protracted unions, but are dissatisfied with those who perform for only a short duration. And this circumstance, some would say, proves that female pleasure is like that of the male.

Sutras 27–31 But this opinion does not hold good, for if it takes a long time to allay a woman's desire, and during this time she is enjoying great pleasure, it is quite natural that she should wish for its continuation. And on this subject there is a verse as follows: "By union with men the lust, desire or passion of women is satisfied, and the pleasure derived from the consciousness of it is called their satisfaction."

Sutras 32–34 Babhravya and his followers say that the semen of women is produced from the beginning of the sexual union and that it continues to be produced until its end, and it is right that it should be so, for if women had no semen there would be no conception.

Sutras 35–36 To this there is an objection. In the beginning of coition the passion of the woman is middling, and she cannot bear the vigorous thrusts of her lover, but by degrees her passion increases until she ceases to think about her body, and then finally she wishes to stop from further coition.

Sutras 37–40 This opinion, however, does not hold good, for just as a potter's wheel, or a top, that revolves with great force does so at first slowly and only gradually becomes very rapid, in the same way the woman's passion begins slowly and increases gradually until she has the desire to discontinue coition, when all the semen has fallen away.

Sutra 41 And there is a verse with regard to this as follows: "The fall of the semen of the man takes place only at the end of coition, while the semen of the woman falls continually, and after the semen of both has all fallen away then they wish for the discontinuance of coition."[4]

Sutras 42–43 Lastly, Vatsyayana is of the opinion that the semen of the female falls in the same way as that of the male.

Now some may ask here: If men and women experience pleasure in much the same way, and since both are engaged in bringing about the same result, why should they have different work to do?

Sutra 44 Vatsya says that this is so because in men and women the ways of working as well as the consciousness of pleasure are different.

Sutras 45–48 How is this? The difference in the ways of working, by which men are the actors and women are the persons acted upon, is owing to the nature of the male active role and the female passive role, otherwise the actor would be sometimes the person acted upon, and vice versa.

Sutra 49 And from this difference in the ways of working follows the difference in the consciousness of pleasure: a man thinks, "this woman is united with me"; and a woman thinks, "I am united with this man".

Sutra 50 It may be said that if the ways of working in men and women are different, why should there not be a difference in the pleasure they feel, which is the result of those ways.

Sutras 51–55 But this objection is groundless; the reason for the difference in their ways of working is because the person acting and the person acted upon are of different kinds. There is no reason for any difference in the pleasure they feel, because they both derive pleasure naturally from the act they perform.[5]

Sutra 56 On this again some may say that when different persons are engaged in doing the same work, we find that they accomplish the same end or purpose; while, on the contrary, in the case of men and women we find that each of them accomplishes his or her own end separately, and this is inconsistent.

Sutras 57–62 But this is a mistake, for we find that sometimes two things are done at the same time; for example, in a ram fight both the rams receive the shock to their heads at the same time. Again, in throwing one wood-apple against another, and also in a fight or struggle of wrestlers. If it be said that in these cases the things employed are of the same kind, it is answered that even in the case of men and women, the nature of the two persons is the same. And as the difference in their ways of working arises from the difference of their conformation only, it follows that men experience the same kind of pleasure as women do.

Sutra 63 There is also a verse on this subject as follows: "Men and women, being of the same nature, feel the same kind of pleasure, and therefore a man should marry such a woman as will love him ever afterwards."

Sutras 64–65 The pleasure of men and women being thus proved to be of the same kind, it follows that, in regard to duration, there are nine kinds of sexual intercourse, in the same way as there are nine kinds according to the force of passion.

Sutra 66 There being thus nine kinds of union with regard to dimensions, force of passion, and duration, respectively, by making combinations of them, innumerable kinds of union would be produced.[6]

Sutra 67 Therefore in each particular kind of sexual union, men should use such means as they may think suitable for the occasion.[7]

Sutras 68–70 At the first time of sexual union the passion of the male is intense, and his duration is short, but in subsequent unions on the same day the reverse of this is the case. With the female, however, it is the contrary, for at the first time her passion is weak, and then her duration long, but on subsequent occasions on the same day, her passion is intense and her duration short, until her passion is satisfied.

Sutra 71 What has been said in this chapter upon the subject of sexual union is sufficient for the learned; but for the edification of the ignorant, the same will now be treated of at length and in detail.

On the different kinds of love

Sutras 72–78 Learned men are of the opinion that love is of four kinds:

Love acquired by continual habit
Love resulting from the imagination
Love resulting from belief
Love resulting from the perception of external objects

Love resulting from the constant and continual performance of some act is called love acquired by constant practice and habit; for example, the love of sexual intercourse, the love of hunting, the love of drinking, the love of gambling, and so on.

Love which is felt for things to which we are not habituated, and which proceeds entirely from ideas, is called love resulting from imagination; for example, that love which some men and women and eunuchs feel for the *auparishtaka* or mouth congress, and that which is felt by all for such things as embracing, kissing, and so on.

The love which is mutual on both sides, and proved to be true, when each looks upon the other as his or her very own, such is called love resulting from belief by the learned.

The love resulting from the perception of external objects is quite evident and well known to the world because the pleasure which it affords is superior to the pleasure of the other kinds of love, which exists only for its sake.

Chapter II Of the embrace

Sutras 1–4 This part of the *Kama Shastra*, which deals with sexual union, is also called "Sixty-four" (*Chatushshashti*). Some say that it is called this because it contains sixty-four chapters. Others are of the opinion that because the author of this part was named Panchala, and the person who recited the part of the *Rig Veda* called *Dashatapa*, which contains sixty-four verses, was also called Panchala, the name "Sixty-four" has been given to the part of the work in honour of the *Rig Veda*s.

Sutra 5 The followers of Babhravya say that this part contains eight subjects: the embrace, kissing, scratching with the nails or fingers, biting, lying down, making various sounds, playing the part of a man, and the *auparishtaka*, or mouth congress. Each of these subjects being of eight kinds, and eight multiplied by eight being sixty-four, this part is therefore named "Sixty-four".

Sutra 6 But Vatsyayana affirms that because this part also contains striking [thrashing], crying, the acts of a man during congress, the various kinds of congress, and other subjects, the name "Sixty-four" is given to it only accidentally. As, for example, we say this tree is seven-leaved (*saptaparna*), or this offering of rice is five-coloured (*panchavarna*), but the tree does not have seven leaves, nor the rice five colours.

Sutras 7–8 Whatever the origins of the sixty-four parts, the embrace, being the first subject, will now be considered. Now the embrace which

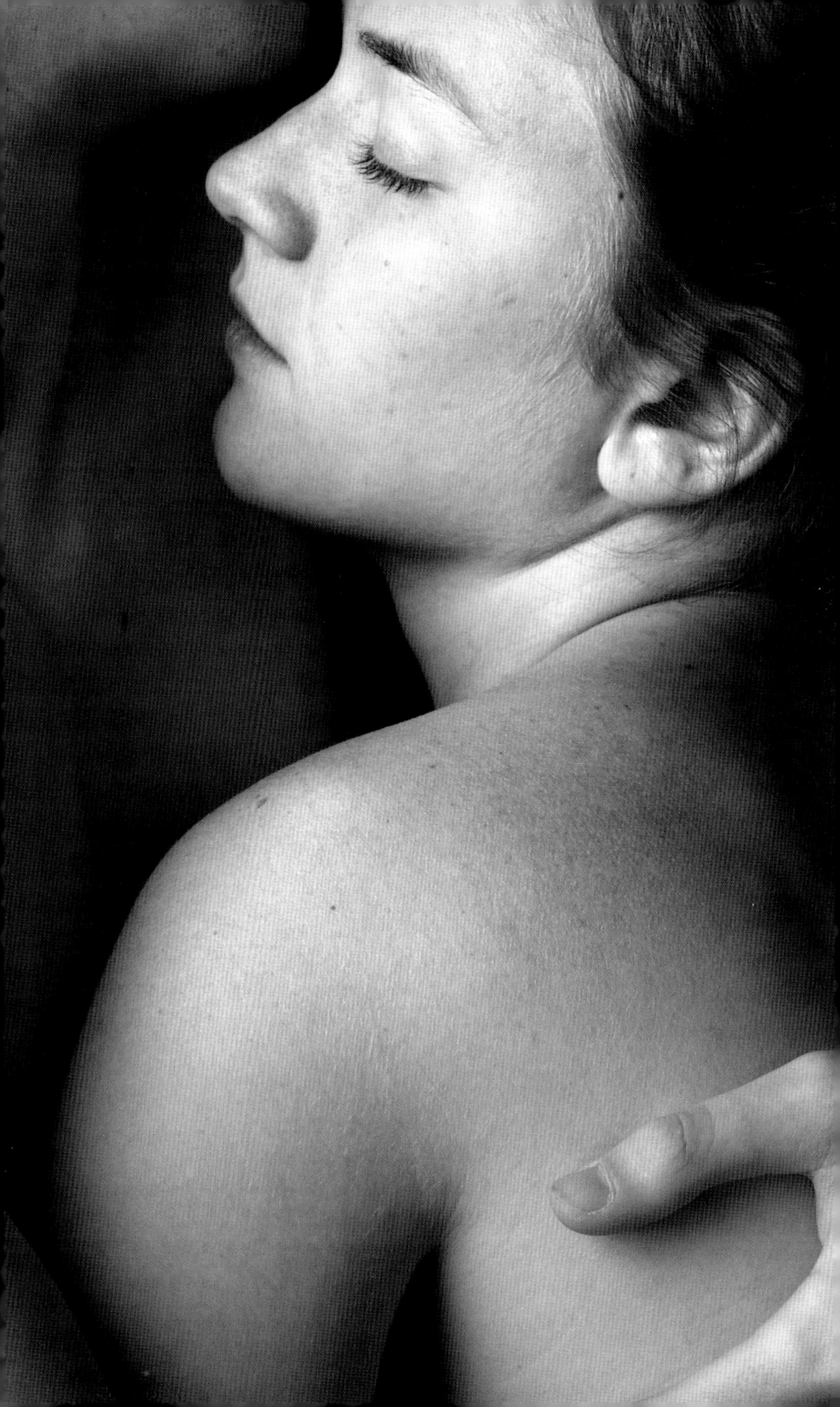

indicates the mutual love of a man and woman who have come together is of four kinds: touching, piercing, rubbing and pressing. The action in each case is denoted by the meaning of the word which stands for it.

Sutra 9 When a man under some pretext or other goes in front of or alongside a woman and touches her body with his own, it is called the "touching embrace".

Sutra 10 When a woman in a lonely place bends down, as if to pick up something, and pierces, as it were, a man sitting or standing, with her breasts, and the man in return takes hold of them, it is called a "piercing embrace".

Sutra 11 These two kinds of embrace take place only between persons who do not, as yet, speak freely with each other.

Sutra 12 When two lovers are walking slowly together, either in the dark, or in a place of public resort, or in a lonely place, and rub their bodies against each other, it is called a "rubbing embrace".

Sutra 13 When on the above occasion one of them presses the other's body forcibly against a wall or pillar, it is called a "pressing embrace".

Sutra 14 These two last embraces are peculiar to those who know the intentions of each other.

Sutra 15 At the time of the union the following four kinds of embrace are used: *Jataveshtitaka*, or the "twining of a creeper"; *Vrikshadhirudhaka*, or "climbing a tree"; *Tila-Tandulaka*, or the "mixture of sesamum seed with rice"; and *Kshiraniraka*, or "milk and water embrace".

Sutra 16 *Jataveshtitaka*: When a woman, clinging to a man as a creeper twines round a tree, bends his head down to hers with the desire of kissing him and slightly makes the sound of "sut sut", embraces him, and looks lovingly toward him, it is called an embrace like the "twining of a creeper".

Sutra 17 *Vrikshadhirudhaka*: When a woman, having placed one of her feet on the foot of her lover, and the other on one of his thighs, passes one of her arms round his back, and the other on his shoulders, makes slightly the sounds of singing and cooing, and wishes, as it were, to climb up him in order to have a kiss, it is called an embrace like the "climbing of a tree".

Sutra 18 Both these kinds of embrace take place when the lovers are standing.

Sutra 19 *Tila-Tandulaka*: When lovers lie on a bed, and embrace each other so closely that the arms and thighs of the one are encircled by the arms and thighs of the other, and are rubbing up against them, this is called an embrace like the "mixture of sesamum seed with rice".

Sutra 20 *Kshiraniraka*: When a man and a woman are very much in love with each other, and, not thinking of any pain or hurt, embrace each other as if they were entering into each other's bodies either while the woman is sitting on the lap of the man, or in front of him, or on a bed, then it is called an embrace like a "mixture of milk and water".

Sutra 21 Both these kinds of embrace take place when both participants feel the urge for sexual union strongly.

Sutra 22 Babhravya has thus related to us the eight kinds of embrace.

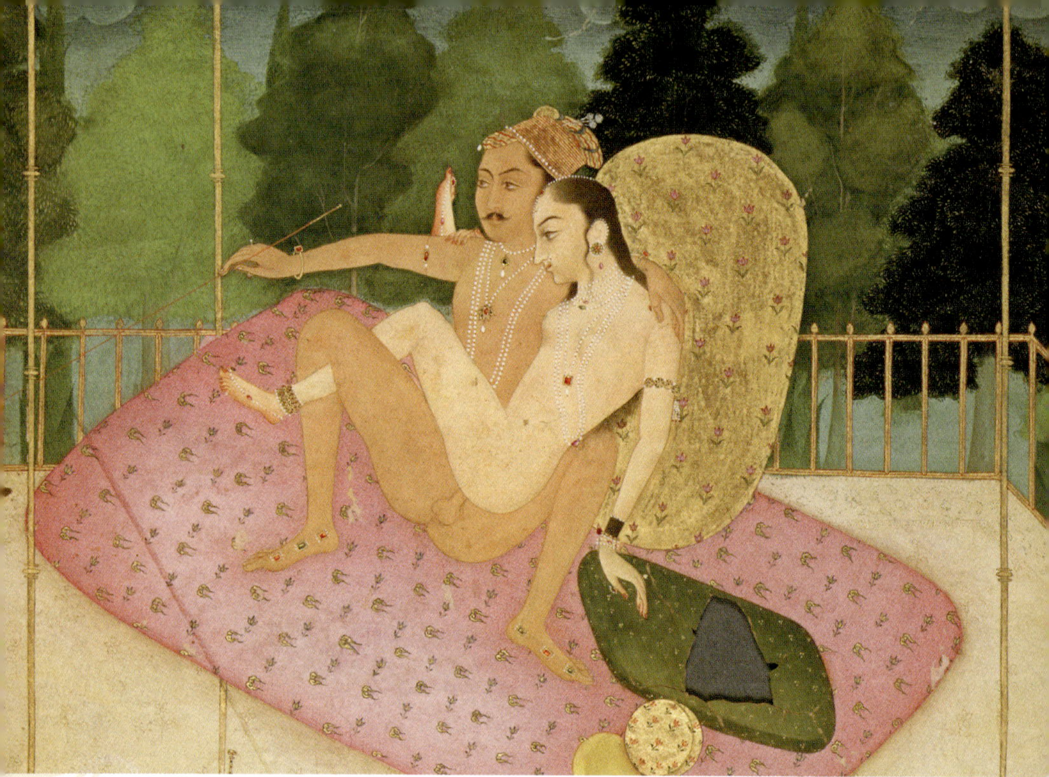

Sutra 23 Suvarnanabha details four ways of embracing parts of the body, which are:

Sutra 24 When one of two lovers presses forcibly one or both of the thighs of the other between his or her own, it is called the "embrace of thighs".

Sutra 25 When a man presses his body against the *jaghana*, or middle part of the woman's body, and mounts upon her to practise, either scratching with the nail or finger, or biting, or striking, or kissing, with the hair of the woman being loose and flowing, it is called the "embrace of the *jaghana*".

Sutra 26 When a man places his chest between the breasts of a woman and presses her with it, it is called the "embrace of the breasts".

Sutra 27 When either of the lovers touches the mouth, the eyes and the forehead of the other with his or her own, it is called the "embrace of the forehead".

Sutra 28 Some say that even shampooing is a kind of embrace, because it involves a mutual touching of bodies.

Sutra 29 But Vatsyayana thinks that shampooing is performed at a different time and for a different purpose, and because it is also of a different character it cannot be said to be an embrace.

Sutra 30 There are also some verses on this subject as follows: "The whole subject of embracing is of such a nature that men who ask questions about it, or who hear about it, or who talk about it, acquire thereby a desire for enjoyment."

Sutra 31 "Even those embraces that are not mentioned in the *Kama Shastra* should be practised at the time of sexual enjoyment if they are in any way conducive to the increase of love or passion."

Sutra 32 "The rules of the *Shastra* apply so long as the passion of the man is middling, but once the wheel of love has been set in motion, there is then no *Shastra* and no order."

Chapter III On kissing

Sutra 1 It is said by some that there is no fixed duration or order of precedence between the embrace, the kiss, and the pressing or scratching with the nails or fingers, and so on.

Sutra 2 Generally, these things should be done before sexual union, while striking and making various sounds accompanies the actual union.

Sutra 3 Vatsyayana, however, thinks that anything may take place at any time, for love does not care for time or order.

Sutra 4 On the occasion of the first congress, kissing and the other things mentioned above should be done moderately, they should not be continued for a long time, and should be done alternately.

Sutra 5 On subsequent occasions, however, the reverse of all this may take place, and moderation will not be necessary, they may continue for a long time, and, for the purpose of kindling love, they may be all done at the same time.

Sutra 6 The proper places for kissing are the following: the forehead, the eyes, the cheeks, the throat, the bosom, the breasts, the lips, and the interior of the mouth.

Sutras 7–8 Moreover the people of Lat [province] also kiss the following places: the joints of the thighs, the arms and the navel. But Vatsyayana thinks that although kissing in the above places is practised by these people on account of the intensity of their love, and the customs of their country, it is not fit to be practised by all.

Sutra 9 In the case of a young girl there are three sorts of kisses: the nominal kiss, the throbbing kiss and the touching kiss.

Sutra 10 When a girl only touches the mouth of her lover with her own, but does not herself do anything, it is called the "nominal kiss".

Sutra 11 When a girl, setting aside her bashfulness a little, wishes to touch the lip that is pressed into her mouth, and with that object moves her lower lip, but not the upper one, it is called the "throbbing kiss".

Sutra 12 When a girl touches her lover's lip with her tongue, and having shut her eyes, places her hands on those of her lover, it is called the "touching kiss".

Sutra 13 Other authors describe four other kinds of kisses: the straight kiss; the bent kiss; the turned kiss; and the pressed kiss.

When the lips of two lovers are brought into direct contact with each other, it is called a "straight kiss".

When the heads of two lovers are bent towards each other, and when so bent, kissing takes place, it is called a "bent kiss".

When one of them turns up the face of the other by holding the head and chin, and then kissing, it is called a "turned kiss".

Lastly, when the lower lip is pressed with much force, it is called a "pressed kiss".

Sutra 14 There is also a fifth kind of kiss called the "greatly pressed kiss", which is effected by taking hold of the lower lip between two fingers, and then, after touching it with the tongue, pressing it with great force with the lip.

Sutras 15–16 As regards kissing, a wager may be laid as to which will get hold of the lips of the other first.

Sutra 17 If the woman loses, she should pretend to cry, should keep her lover off by shaking her hands, and turn away from him and dispute with him saying, "let another wager be laid". If she loses this a second time, she should appear doubly distressed.

Sutra 18 When her lover is off his guard or asleep, she should get hold of his lower lip, and hold it in her teeth, so that it should not slip away, and then she should laugh, make a loud noise, deride him, dance about, and say whatever she likes in a joking way, moving her eyebrows and rolling her eyes.

Sutra 19 Such are the wagers and quarrels as far as kissing is concerned, but the same may be applied with regard to the pressing or scratching with the nails and fingers, biting and striking.

Sutra 20 All these, however, are peculiar to men and women of intense passion.

Sutra 21 When a man kisses the upper lip of a woman, while she in return kisses his lower lip, it is called the "kiss of the upper lip".

Sutra 22 When one of them takes both the lips of the other between his or her own, it is called "a clasping kiss". A woman, however, only takes this kind of kiss from a man without a moustache.

Sutra 23 And on the occasion of this kiss, if one of them touches the teeth, the tongue and the palate of the other, with his or her tongue, it is called the "fighting of the tongue".

Sutra 24 In the same way, the pressing of the teeth of the one against the mouth of the other is to be practised.

Sutra 25 Kissing is of four kinds: moderate, contracted, pressed and soft, according to the different parts of the body which are kissed, because different kinds of kisses are appropriate for different parts of the body.

Sutra 26 When a woman looks at the face of her lover while he is asleep and kisses it to show her intention or desire, it is called a "kiss that kindles love".

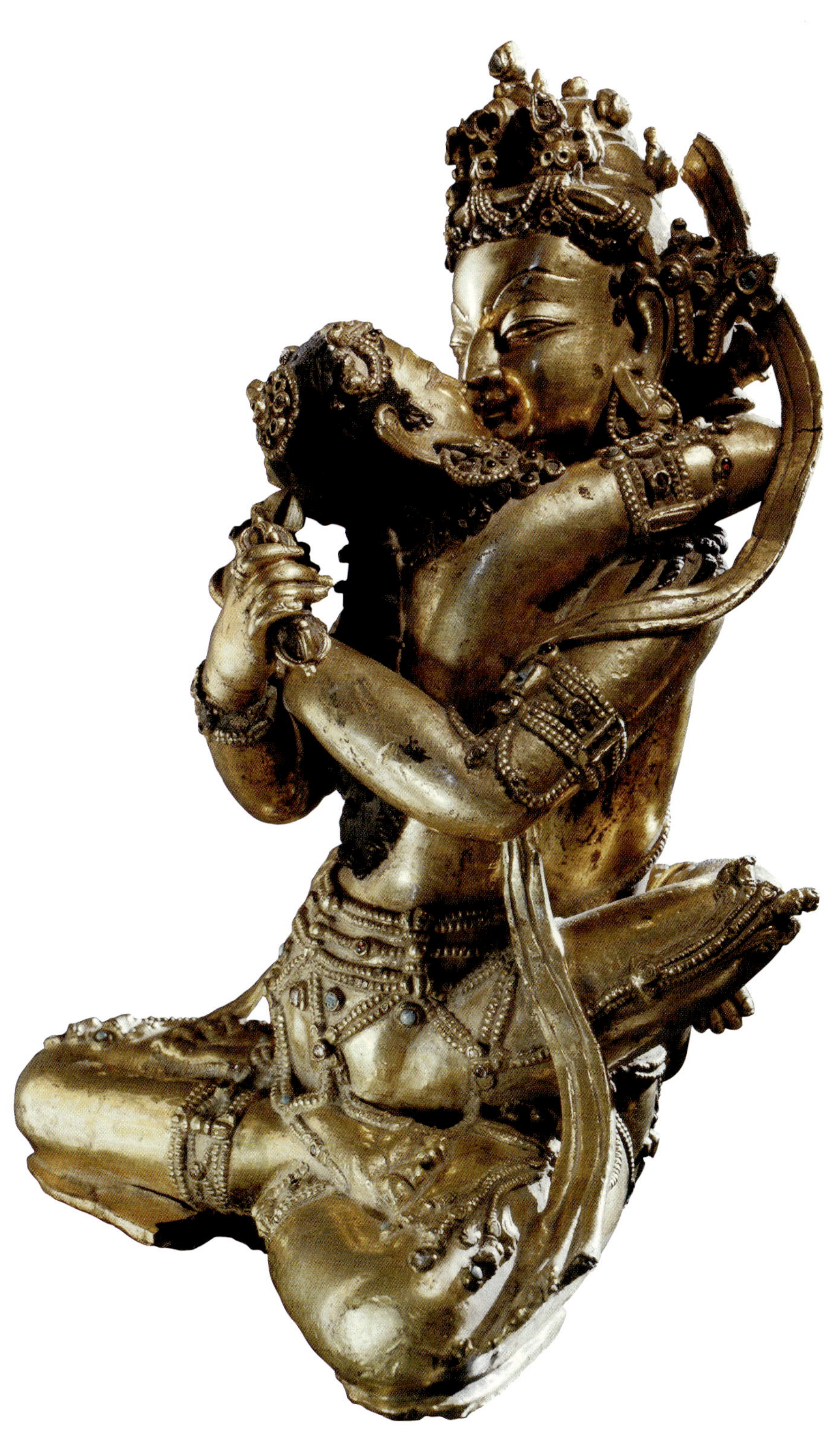

Sutra 27 When a woman kisses her lover while he is engaged in business, or while he is quarrelling with her, or while he is looking at something else, so that his mind may be turned away, it is called a "kiss that turns away".

Sutra 28 When a lover, returning home late at night, kisses his beloved, who is asleep on her bed, in order to show her his desire, it is called a "kiss that awakens".

Sutra 29 On such an occasion the woman may pretend to be asleep at the time of her lover's arrival, so that she may know his intention and obtain respect from him.

Sutra 30 When a person kisses the reflection of the person he loves in a mirror, in water or on a wall, it is called a "kiss showing the intention".

Sutra 31 When a person kisses a child sitting on his lap, or a picture, or an image or figure, in the presence of the person beloved by him, it is called a "transferred kiss".

Sutras 32–33 When a man coming up to a woman, at night at a theatre or in a family gathering, kisses the fingers of the hand, or when a woman is shampooing or massaging her lover's body and places her face on his thigh (as if she was sleepy) so as to inflame his passion, or kisses his thigh or great toe, it is called a "demonstrative kiss".

Sutra 34 There is also a verse on this subject as follows: "Whatever things may be done by one of the lovers to the other, it should be reciprocated." For example, if the woman kisses him, he should kiss her in return; if she strikes him, he should strike her in return – each gesture to be returned with equal intensity.

Chapter IV On marking with the nails

Sutra 1 When love becomes intense, pressing with the nails or scratching the body with them is practised.

Sutras 2–3 It is done on the following occasions: on the first union, when setting out on a journey, on the return from a journey, when an angry lover is reconciled, and lastly when the woman is intoxicated.

But pressing with the nails or biting is not a usual thing, being agreeable only to those who are full of passion.

Sutra 4 Pressing with the nails is of the eight following kinds, according to the forms of the marks which are produced: a "sounding", a "half moon", a "circle", a "line", a "tiger's nail" or "claw", a "peacock's foot", the "jump of a hare" and the "leaf of a blue lotus".

Sutra 5 The places that are to be pressed with the nails are as follows: the armpit, the throat, the breasts, the lips, the *jaghana*, or middle parts of the body, and the thighs.

Sutras 6–7 But Suvarnanabha maintains that when the impetuosity of passion is excessive, it need not be considered where the nails are placed.

Sutra 8 The qualities of good nails are that they should be bright, well set, clean, entire, convex, soft, and glossy in appearance. Nails are of three kinds according to their size: small, middling and large.

Sutra 9 Large nails, which give grace to the hands, and attract the hearts of women from their appearance, are possessed by the Bengalis.

Sutra 10 Small nails, which can be used in various ways, and are to be

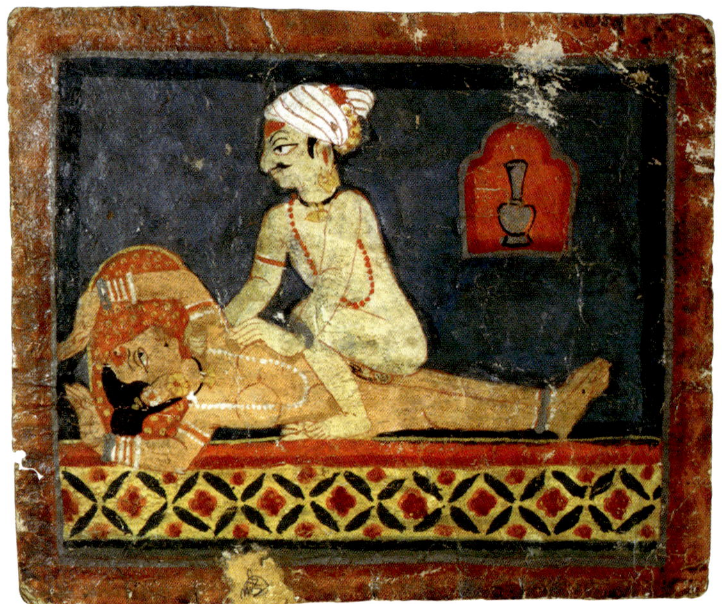

applied only with the object of giving pleasure, are possessed by the people of the southern districts.

Sutra 11 Middling nails, which contain the properties of both the above kinds, belong to the people of the Maharashtra.

Sutras 12–13 When a person presses the chin, the breasts, the lower lip or the *jaghana* of another so softly that no scratch or mark is left, but only the hair on the body becomes erect from the touch of the nails, and the nails themselves make a sound, it is called a "sounding" or pressing with the nails.

This pressing is used in the case of a young girl when her lover shampoos her, scratches her head and wants to trouble or frighten her.

Sutra 14 The curved mark with the nails, which is impressed on the neck and the breasts, is called the "half moon".

Sutras 15–16 When the "half moons" are impressed opposite to each other, it is called a "circle". This mark with the nails is generally made on the navel, the small cavities about the buttocks and on the joints of the thigh.

Sutra 17 A mark in the form of a small line, and which can be made on any part of the body, is called a "line".

Sutra 18 This same line, when it is curved, and made on the breast, is called a "tiger's nail".

Sutra 19 When a curved mark is made on the breast by means of the five nails, it is called a "peacock's foot". This mark is made to elicit praise, for it requires a great deal of skill to make it properly.

Sutra 20 When five marks with the nails are made close to one another near the nipple of the breast, it is called "the jump of a hare".

Sutra 21 A mark made on the breast or on the hips in the form of a leaf of the blue lotus is called the "leaf of a blue lotus".

Sutra 22 When a person is going on a journey and makes a mark on the thighs, or on the breast, it is called a "token of remembrance". On such an occasion three or four lines are impressed close to one another with the nails.

Sutra 23 Here ends the marking with the nails. Marks of many other kinds than the above may also be made with the nails.

Sutra 24 As the ancient authors say, there are innumerable degrees of skill among men (the practice of this art being known to all), so there are innumerable ways of making these marks. And as pressing or marking with the nails is independent of love, no one can say with certainty how many different kinds of nail marks actually exist.

Sutra 25 The reason for this, Vatsyayana says, is that as variety is necessary in love, so love is to be produced by means of variety. It is on this account that courtesans, who are well acquainted with various ways and means, become so desirable, for if variety is sought in all the arts and amusements, such as archery and others, how much more should it be sought after in the science of love.

Sutra 26 The marks of the nails should not be made on the body of a married women, but particular kinds of marks may be made on their private parts for the sake of remembrance and the increase of love.

Sutras 27–28 There are also some verses on the subject, as follows: "The love of a woman who sees nail marks on the private parts of her body, even though they are old and almost worn out, becomes fresh and renewed. Without nail marks to remind a person of the passages of love, love is lessened in the same way as when no union takes place for a long time."

Sutra 29 Even when a stranger sees at a distance a young woman with the marks of nails on her breast,[8] he is filled with love and respect for her.

Sutra 30 In the same way, a man who carries the marks of nails and teeth on some parts of his body influences the mind of a woman, even though it be ever so firm.

Sutra 31 In short, nothing tends to increase love so much as the effects of marking with the nails, and biting.

Chapter V On biting

Sutra 1 All the places that can be kissed are also the places that can be bitten, except the upper lip, the interior of the mouth and the eyes.

Sutra 2 Good teeth should have the following qualities: they should be equal, possessed of a pleasing brightness, capable of being coloured, of proper proportions, unbroken and with sharp ends.

Sutra 3 Defective teeth are blunt, protruding from the gums, rough, soft, large and loosely set.

Sutras 4–19 The different kinds of biting are as follows: the hidden bite, the swollen bite, the point, the line of points, the coral and the jewel, the line of jewels, the broken cloud and the biting of the boar.

The "hidden bite" is biting that shows only because of the excessive redness of the skin that is bitten.

The "swollen bite" is when the skin is pressed down on both sides.

The "point" is when a small portion of the skin is bitten with two teeth only.

The "line of points" is when such small portions of the skin are bitten with all the teeth.

The "coral and the jewel" is biting which is done by bringing together the teeth and the lips. The lip is the coral, and the teeth the jewel.

The "line of jewels" is when biting is done with all the teeth.

The "broken cloud" is biting which consists of unequal risings in a circle, and which comes from the space between the teeth. This is impressed on the breasts.

The "biting of a boar" consists of many broad rows of marks near to one another, and with red intervals. This is impressed on the breasts and the shoulders; and these two last modes of biting are peculiar to persons of intense passion.

The lower lip is the place on which the "hidden bite", the "swollen bite" and the "point" are made; again, the "swollen bite" and the "coral and the jewel" bite are done on the cheek. Kissing, pressing with the nails and biting are the ornaments of the left cheek, and when the word cheek is used it is to be understood as the left one.

Both the "line of points" and the "line of jewels" are to be impressed on the throat, the armpit and the joints of the thighs; but the "line of points" alone is to be impressed on the forehead and the thighs.

The marking with the nails and the biting of the following things – an ornament of the forehead, an ear ornament, a bunch of flowers, a betel leaf or a tamala leaf, which are worn by, or belong to, the woman that is beloved – are signs of the desire of enjoyment.

Here ends the different kinds of biting.

Sutra 20 In the affairs of love a man should do such things as are agreeable to the women of different countries.

Sutra 21 The women of the central countries (that is, between the Ganges and the Jumna) are noble in their character, not accustomed to disgraceful practices and dislike pressing the nails and biting.

Sutras 22–23 The women of Bahlika and Avanti hate kissing, marking with the nails and biting, but they have a fondness for various kinds of sexual union.

Sutra 24 The women of Malwa and Abhira like embracing and kissing, but not wounding, and they are gained over by striking.

Sutra 25 The women about the Indus and five rivers (that is, the Punjab), are gained over by the *auparishtaka* or mouth congress.

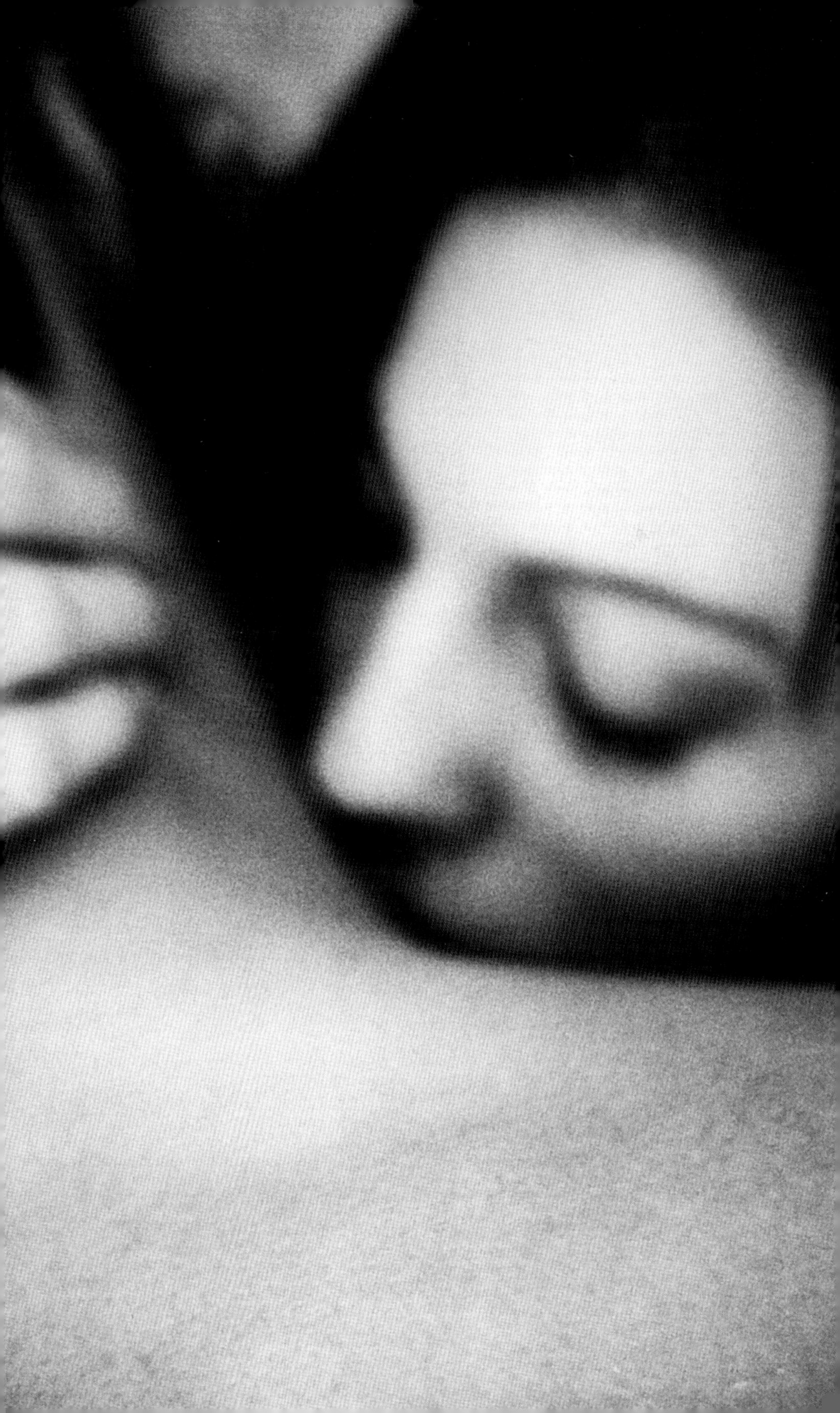

Sutra 26 The women of Aparatika and the Lat country are full of passion, and slowly make the sound "Sit".

Sutra 27 The women of Strirajya and Koshola (Oude) are also full of impetuous desire. Their semen falls in large quantities and they are fond of "taking medicine"[9] to make it do so.

Sutra 28 The women of the Andhra country have tender bodies, are fond of enjoyment and have a liking for voluptuous pleasures.

Sutra 29 The women of Maharashtra are fond of practising the sixty-four arts; they utter low and harsh words, like to be spoken to in the same way, and have an impetuous desire of enjoyment.

Sutra 30 The women of Pataliputra (that is, modern Patna) are of the same nature as the women of Maharashtra, but they reveal their likings only in secret.

Sutra 31 The women of the Dravida country [South India], despite being rubbed and pressed at the time of sexual enjoyment, have a slow fall of semen – that is, they are very slow in the act of coition.

Sutra 32 The women of Vanavasi are moderately passionate, and while they go through every kind of enjoyment, they cover their bodies and abuse those who utter low, mean and harsh words.

Sutra 33 The women of Gauda have tender bodies and speak sweetly.

Sutra 34 Now, Suvarnanabha is of the opinion that that which is agreeable to the nature of a particular person is of more consequence than that which is agreeable to a whole nation, and that therefore the peculiarities of the country should not be observed in such cases.

Sutra 35 In time the various pleasures, dress and sports of one country are borrowed by another, and in such a case these things must be considered as belonging originally to that country.

Sutra 36 Among the things mentioned earlier – embracing, kissing, and so on – those which increase passion should be done first, and those which are only for amusement or variety should be done afterwards.

Sutra 37 There is a verse on this subject: "When a man bites a woman forcibly, she should angrily do the same to him with double force."

Sutra 38 In retaliating, a "point" should be returned with a "line of points", and a "line of points" with a "broken cloud", and if she be excessively chafed, she should at once begin a love quarrel with him.

Sutra 39 At such a time she should take hold of her lover by the hair, and bend his head down, and kiss his lower lip.

Sutra 40 Then, being intoxicated with love, she should shut her eyes and bite him in various places.

Sutras 41–42 Even by day, and in a place of public resort, when her lover shows her any mark that she may have inflicted on his body, she should smile at the sight of it. Turning her face as if she were going to chide him, she should, with an angry look, show him the marks on her own body that he has made.

Sutra 43 Thus, if men and women act according to each other's liking, their love for each other will not be lessened even in 100 years.

Chapter VI The various kinds of congress

Sutras 1–2 When uniting in a "high congress" the deer woman (*mrigi*) should lie down in such a way as to widen her *yoni*, while in a "low congress" the elephant woman (*hastini*) should lie down so as to contract her *yoni*. But in an "equal congress" the woman should lie down in the natural position.

Sutras 3–6 What is said above concerning the deer woman and the elephant woman applies also to the mare woman (*vadawa*). In a "low congress" the woman should particularly make use of medicine, to cause her desires to be satisfied quickly.

Sutra 7 The deer woman has the following three ways of lying down: the "widely opened position", the "yawning position" and the "position of the wife of Indra".

Sutras 8–9 When she lowers her head and raises her middle parts it is called the "widely opened position". At such a time the man should apply some unguent, so as to make the entrance easy.

Sutra 10 When she raises her thighs and keeps them wide apart and engages in congress, it is called the "yawning position".

Sutras 11–12 When she places her thighs with her legs doubled on them upon her sides, and thus engages in congress, it is called the "position of Indrani" and this is learned only by practice. The position is also useful in the case of the "highest congress".

Sutras 13–14 The "clasping position" is used in "low congress", and should be used by the elephant woman in the "lowest congress", together with the "pressing position", the "twining position" and the "mare's position".

Sutra 15 The "clasping position" is when, during congress, the legs of both the male and the female are stretched straight out over each other.

Sutras 16–17 It is of two kinds, the "side position" and the "supine position", according to the way in which they lie down. In the "side position" the male should invariably lie on his left side, and cause the woman to lie on her right side, and this rule is to be observed in lying down with all kinds of women.

Sutra 18 The "pressing position" is when, after congress has begun in the "clasping position", the woman presses her lover with her thighs.

Sutra 19 The "twining position" is when the woman places one of her thighs across the thigh of her lover.

Sutra 20 The "mare's position" is when a woman forcibly holds the *lingam* in her *yoni* after it is in.

This is learned only by much practice and is chiefly found among the women of the Andhra country.

Sutra 21 The above are the seven different positions mentioned by Babhravya. Suvarnanabha, however, gives the following in addition:

Sutra 22 When the female raises both of her thighs straight up, it is called the "rising position".

Sutra 23 When she raises both of her legs and places them on her lover's shoulders, it is called the "yawning position".

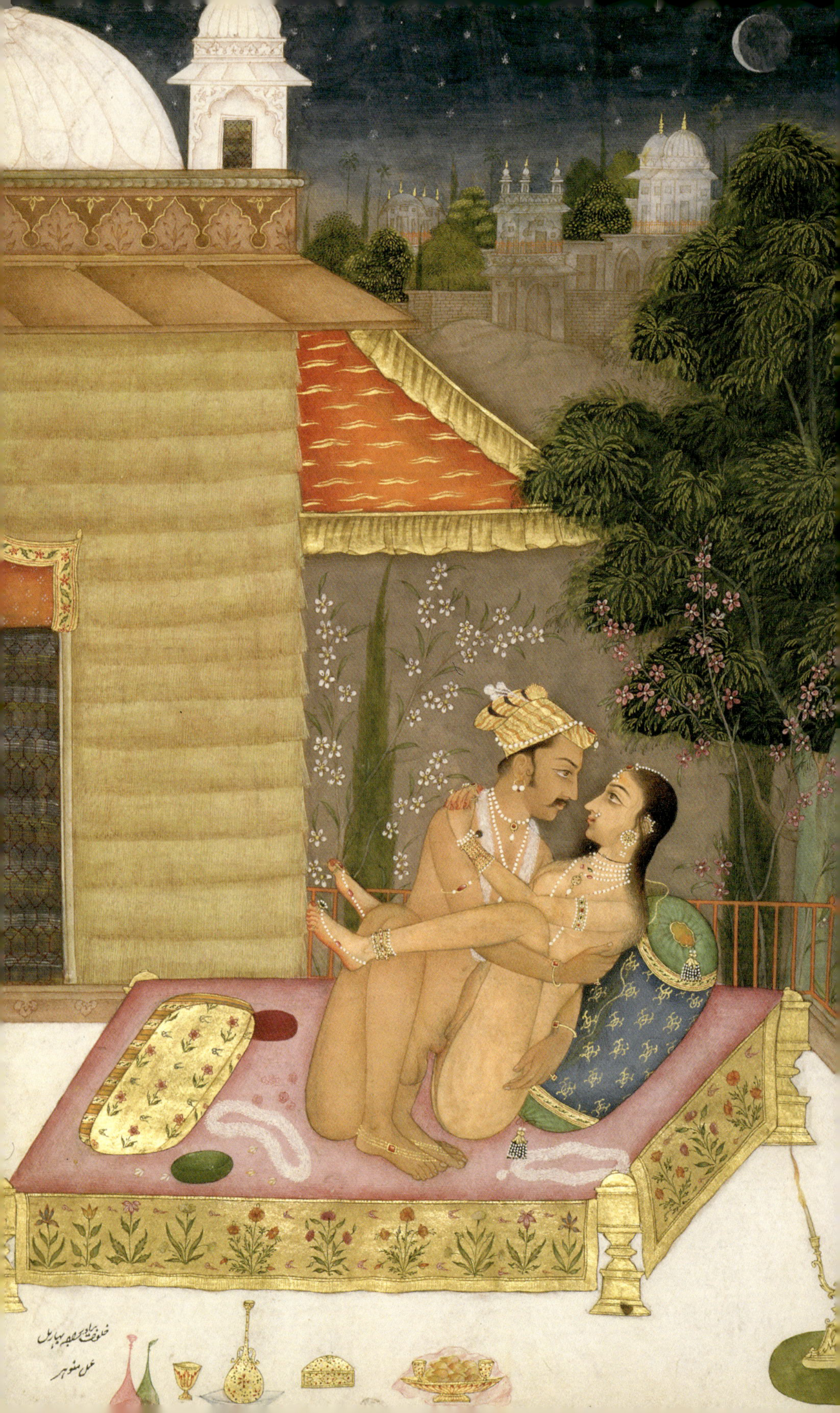

عمل منوهر

Sutra 24 When the legs are contracted, and thus held by the lover before his bosom, it is called the "pressed position".

Sutra 25 When only one of her legs is stretched out, it is called the "half-pressed position".

Sutra 26 When the woman places one of her legs on her lover's shoulder, and stretches the other out, and then places the latter on his shoulder, and stretches out the other, and continues to do so alternately, it is called the "splitting of a bamboo".

Sutra 27 When one of her legs is placed on the head and the other is stretched out, it is called the "fixing of a nail". This is learned only by much practice.

Sutra 28 When both the legs of the woman are contracted and placed on her stomach, it is called the "crab's position".

Sutra 29 When the thighs are raised and placed one upon the other, it is called the "packed position".

Sutra 30 When the shanks are placed one upon the other, it is called the "lotus-like position".

Sutra 31 When a man, during congress, turns round and enjoys the woman without leaving her, while she embraces him round the back all the time, it is called the "turning position", and is learned only by practice.

Sutras 32–34 Thus, says Suvarnanabha, these different ways of lying down, sitting and standing should be practised in water, because it is easy to do so therein. But Vatsyayana is of the opinion that congress in water is improper, because it is prohibited by the religious law.

Sutra 35 When a man and a woman support themselves on each other's bodies, or on a wall or pillar, and thus engage in congress while standing, it is called the "supported congress".

Sutra 36 When a man supports himself against a wall, and the woman, sitting on his hands joined together and held underneath her, throws her arms round his neck, and putting her thighs alongside his waist, moves herself by her feet, which are touching the wall against which the man is leaning, it is called the "suspended congress".

Sutra 37 When a woman stands on her hands and feet like a quadruped, and her lover mounts her like a bull, it is called the "congress of a cow".

Sutra 38 At this time everything that is ordinarily done on the bosom should be done on the back.

Sutra 39 In the same way a man and woman can carry on the "congress of a dog", the "congress of a goat", the "congress of a deer", the "forcible mounting of an ass", the "congress of a cat", the "jump of a tiger", the "pressing of an elephant", the "rubbing of a boar" and the "mounting of a horse".

And in all these cases the characteristics of these different animals should be manifested by acting like them.

Sutra 40 When a man unites with two women at the same time, both of whom love him in equal measure, it is called the "united congress".

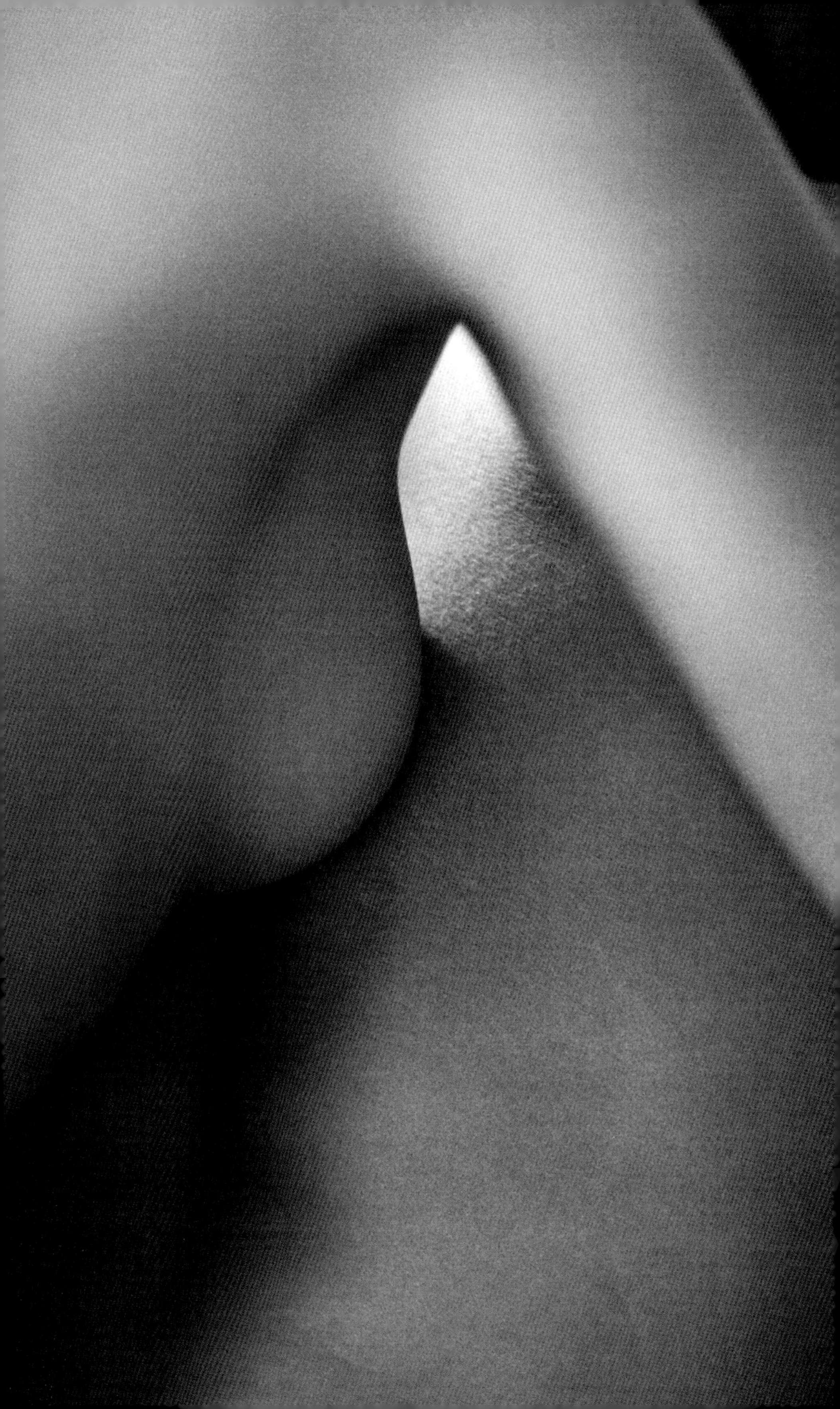

Sutra 41 When a man enjoys many women altogether, it is called the "congress of a herd of cows".

Sutra 42 The following kinds of congress – sporting in water, or the congress of an elephant with many female elephants, which is said to take place only in a water pool; the congress of a collection of goats; the congress of a collection of deer – take place in imitation of these animals.

Sutra 43 In Gramaneri many young men enjoy one woman, either one after the other, or at the same time.

Sutra 44 Thus one of them holds her, another enjoys her, a third uses her mouth, a fourth holds her middle part, and in this way they go on enjoying her several parts alternately.

Sutra 45 The same things can be done when several men are sitting in company with one courtesan, or when one courtesan is alone with many men. In the same way this can be done by the women of the king's harem when they accidentally get hold of a man.

Sutras 46–47 The people in the Southern countries also have a congress in the anus that is called the "lower congress".

Sutras 48–49 Thus ends the various kinds of congress. There are also two verses on the subject as follows: "An ingenious person should multiply the kinds of congress after the fashion of the different kinds of beasts and of birds. For these different kinds of congress, performed according to the usage of each country, and the liking of each individual, generate love, friendship and respect in the hearts of women."

Chapter VII The various modes of thrashing, and the sounds appropriate to them

Sutra 1 Sexual intercourse can be compared to a quarrel, on account of the inconsistencies of love and its tendency to dispute.

Sutra 2 In a state of ardour, striking or thrashing is considered one of the factors for arousing passion, and on the body the special places are the shoulders, the head, the space between the breasts, the back, the *jaghana*, or middle part of the body, and the sides.

Sutra 3 Striking is of four kinds: striking with the back of the hand, striking with the fingers a little contracted, striking with the fist and striking with the open palm of the hand.

Sutras 4–5 On account of its causing pain, striking gives rise to shrieking, which is of various kinds, and to the eight kinds of crying:

Sutra 6 The inarticulate sound *hin*, the thundering sound, the cooing sound, the weeping sound, the sound *phut*, the sound *phat*, the sound *sut* and the sound *plat*.

Sutras 7–8 Besides these, there are also words having a meaning, such as "mother", and those that are expressive of prohibition, sufficiency, desire of liberation, pain or praise, and to which may be added sounds like those of the dove, the cuckoo, the green pigeon, the parrot, the bee, the sparrow, the flamingo, the duck and the quail, which are all occasionally made use of.

Sutras 9–10 Blows with the fist should be given on the back of the woman while she is sitting on the lap of the man, and she should give

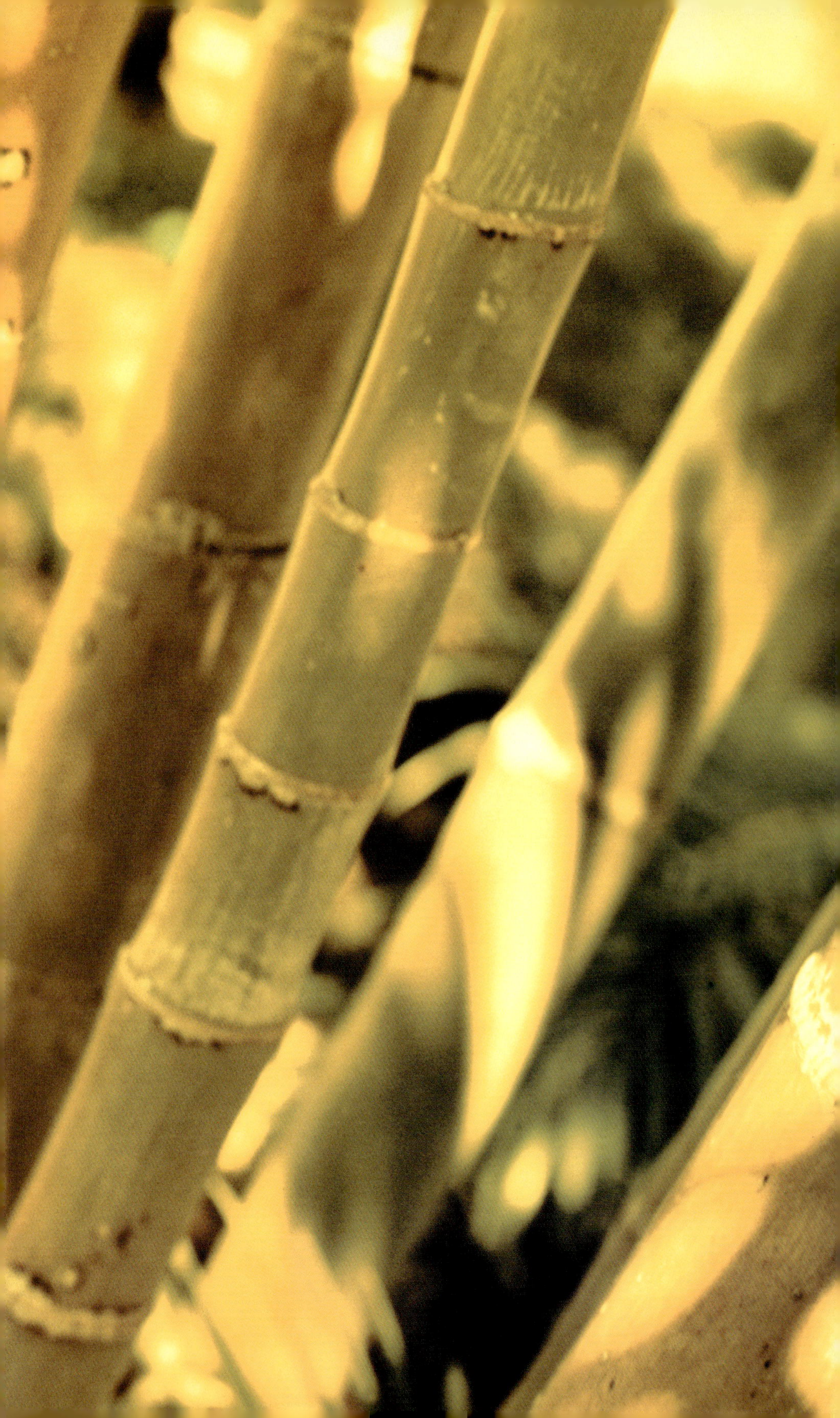

blows in return, abusing the man as if she were angry, and making the cooing and the weeping sounds.

Sutras 11–12 While the woman is engaged in congress the space between the breasts should be struck with the back of the hand, slowly at first, and then proportionately to the increasing excitement, until the end.

Sutra 13 At this time the sound *hin* and others may be made, alternately or optionally, according to habit.

Sutra 14 When the man, making the sound *phat*, strikes the woman on the head, with the fingers of his hand a little contracted, it is called *prasritaka*.

Sutras 15–16 At that time the appropriate sounds are the cooing sound, the sound *phat* and the sound *phut* inside the mouth, and at the end of congress the sighing and weeping sounds. *Phat* is an imitation of the sound of a bamboo being split.

Sutra 17 *Phut* is like the sound made by something falling into water.

Sutra 18 At all times when kissing and such things are begun, the woman should reply with a hissing sound.

Sutras 19–20 During the excitement when the woman is not accustomed to striking, she continually utters words expressive of prohibition, of having had sufficient, or desiring to be set free, as well as the words "father" and "mother", intermingled with the sighing, weeping and thundering sounds.[10] Toward the conclusion of the congress, the breasts, the *jaghana* and the sides of the woman should be pressed with the open palms of the hand, with some force, until the end of it and and then sounds like those of the quail or the goose should be made.

Sutra 21 There are two verses on the subject as follows:

"The characteristics of manhood are said to consist of roughness and impetuosity, while weakness, tenderness, sensibility and an inclination to turn away from unpleasant things are those of womanhood."

Sutra 22 "The excitement of passion and peculiarities of habit may sometimes cause contrary results to appear, but these do not last long, and in the end the natural state is resumed."

Sutra 23 The "wedge on the bosom", the "scissors on the head", the "piercing instrument on the cheeks" and the "pinchers on the breasts and sides", may also be taken into consideration with the other four modes of striking, and thus give eight ways altogether. But these four ways of striking with instruments are peculiar to the people of the southern countries, and the marks caused by them are seen on the breasts of their women.

Sutra 24 Vatsyayana is of the opinion that the practice of them is painful, barbarous and base, and quite unworthy of imitation.

Sutra 25 In the same way, anything that is a local peculiarity should not always be adopted elsewhere.

Sutra 26 Even in the place where a practice is prevalent, excess of it should always be avoided.

Sutra 27 The king of the Panchalas killed the courtesan Madhavasena by means of the wedge during congress.

Sutra 28 Satakarni Satavahana of the Kuntalas deprived his great queen Malayavati of her life with a pair of scissors.

Sutra 29 Naradeva, whose hand was deformed, blinded a dancing girl by directing a piercing instrument in a wrong way.

Sutra 30 There are two verses on the subject as follows:

"About these things there cannot be either enumeration or any definite rule. Congress having once commenced, passion alone gives birth to all the acts of the parties."

Sutra 31 "Such passionate actions and amorous gesticulations or movements, which arise on the spur of the moment, and during sexual intercourse, cannot be defined and are as elusive as dreams."

Sutras 32–33 Having attained the fifth degree of motion a horse goes on with blind speed, regardless of pits, ditches and posts in its way; and in the same manner a loving pair become blind with passion in the heat of congress, and they go on with great impetuosity, paying not the least regard to excess.

Sutra 34 For this reason, one who is well acquainted with the science of love, and knowing his own strength, as well as the tenderness, impetuosity and strength of the young woman, should act accordingly.

Sutra 35 The various modes of enjoyment are not for all times or for all persons, but should only be used at the proper time and in the proper countries and places.

Chapter VIII About women acting the part of a man; and the work of a man

Sutra 1 When a woman sees that her lover is fatigued by constant congress, without having his desire satisfied, she should, with his permission, lay him down upon his back, and give him assistance by acting his part. She may also do this to satisfy the curiosity of her lover, or her own desire of novelty.

Sutra 2 There are two ways of doing this: the first is when during congress she turns round, and gets on top of her lover, in such a manner as to continue the congress, without obstructing the pleasure of it; and the other is when she acts the man's part from the beginning.

Sutra 3 At such a time, with flowers in her loose-hanging hair, and her smiles broken by hard breathing, pressing upon her lover's bosom with her own breasts, and lowering her head frequently, she should retaliate with all the same actions her lover used on her before, returning his blows and chafing him, saying, "I was laid down by you, and fatigued with hard congress; I shall now therefore lay you down in return". She should then, fatigued, display her bashfulness and show that she desires to end the congress. In this way she should do the work of a man, which we shall presently relate.

Sutra 4 What follows is whatever is done by a man to give pleasure to a woman, and is called "the work of a man".

Sutra 5 While the woman is lying on his bed, and is, as it were, abstracted by his conversation, he should loosen the knot of her undergarments, and when she begins to dispute with him, he should overwhelm her with kisses. Then when his *lingam* is erect he should

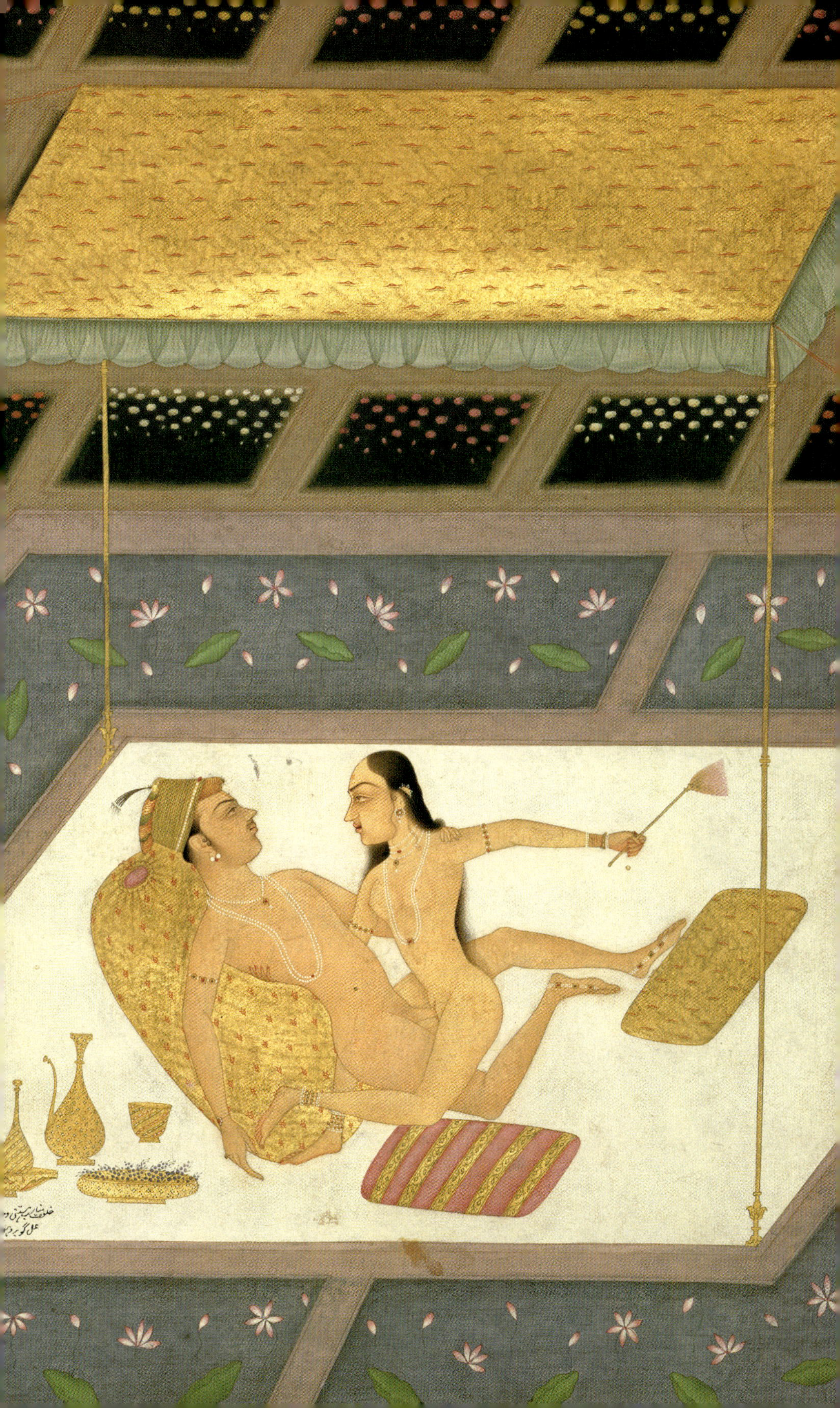

touch her with his hands in various places, and gently manipulate various parts of the body. If the woman is bashful, and if it is the first time that they have come together, the man should place his hands between her thighs, which she would probably keep close together, and if she is a very young girl, he should first get his hands upon her breasts, which she would probably cover with her own hands, and under her armpits and on her neck. If however she is a seasoned woman, he should do whatever is agreeable either to him or to her, and whatever is fitting for the occasion. After this he should take hold of her hair and hold her chin in his fingers for the purpose of kissing her. Upon this, if she is a young girl, she will become bashful and close her eyes.

Sutra 6 In any case, he should gather from the action of the woman what things would be pleasing to her during congress.

Sutra 7 Here Suvarnanabha says that while a man is doing to the woman what he likes best during congress, he should always make a point of pressing those parts of her body on which she turns her eyes.

Sutra 8 The signs of the enjoyment and satisfaction of the woman are as follows: her body relaxes, she closes her eyes, she puts aside all bashfulness, and shows increased willingness to unite the two organs as closely together as possible.

Sutra 9 On the other hand, the signs of her want of enjoyment and of failing to be satisfied are as follows: she shakes her hands, she does not let the man get up, feels dejected, bites the man, kicks him, and continues to go on moving after the man has finished.

Sutra 10 In such cases the man should rub the *yoni* of the woman with his hand and fingers (as the elephant rubs anything with his trunk) before engaging in congress, until it is softened, and after that is done he should proceed to put his *lingam* into her.

Sutra 11 The acts to be done by the man are: "moving forward", "friction" or "churning", "piercing", "rubbing", "pressing", "giving a blow", the "blow of a boar", the "blow of a bull", the "sporting of a sparrow".

Sutra 12 When the organs are brought together properly and directly it is called "moving the organ forward".

Sutra 13 When the *lingam* is held with the hand, and turned all round in the *yoni*, it is called "churning".

Sutra 14 When the *yoni* is lowered, and the upper part of it is struck with the *lingam*, it is called "piercing".

Sutra 15 When the same thing is done on the lower part of the *yoni*, it is called "rubbing".

Sutra 16 When the *yoni* is pressed by the *lingam* for a long time, it is called "pressing".

Sutra 17 When the *lingam* is removed to some distance from the *yoni*, and then forcibly strikes it, it is called "giving a blow".

Sutra 18 When only one part of the *yoni* is rubbed with the *lingam*, it is called the "blow of a boar".

Sutra 19 When both sides of the *yoni* are rubbed in this way, it is called the "blow of a bull".

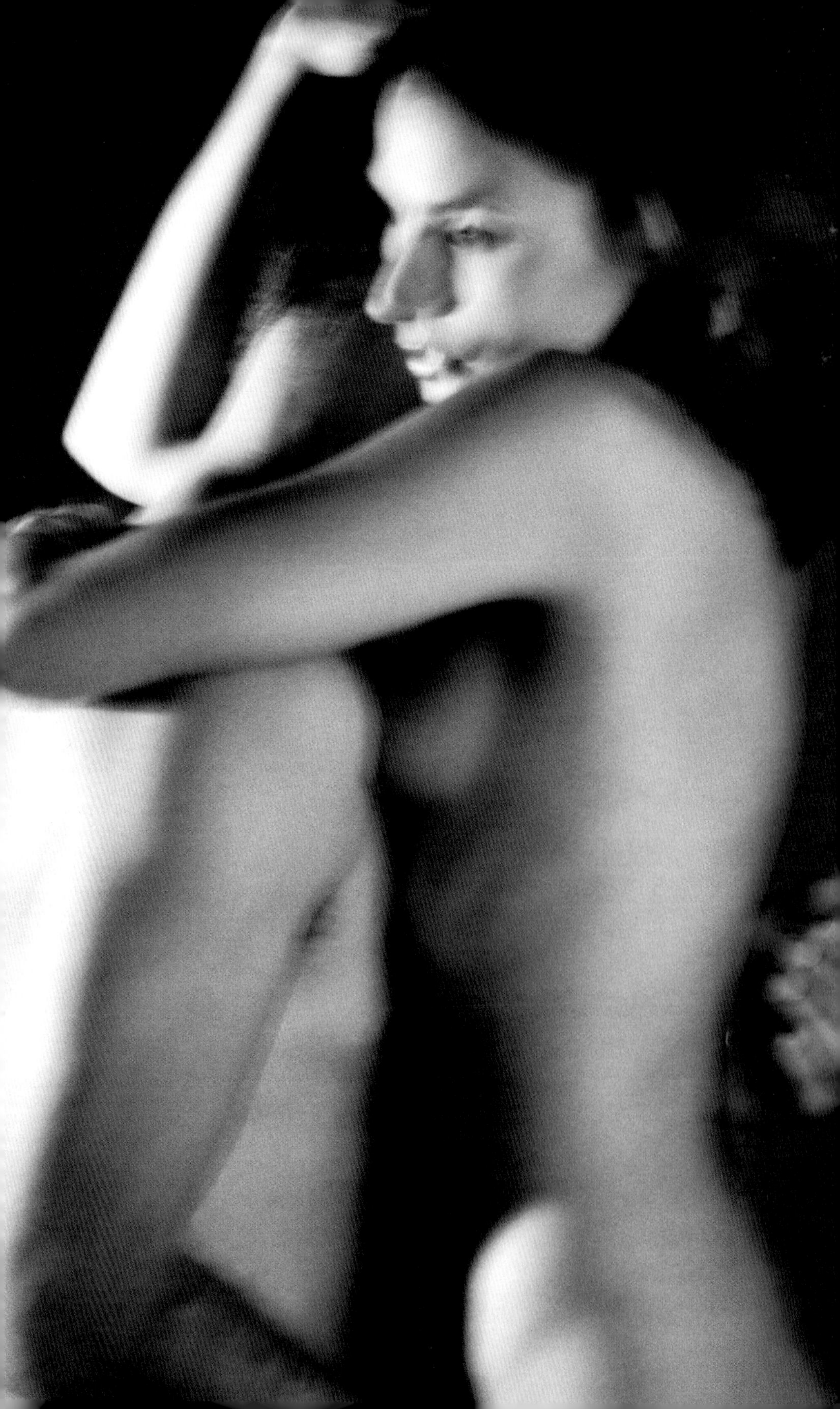

Sutras 20–22 When the *lingam* is in the *yoni*, and moved up and down frequently, and without being taken out, it is called the "sporting of a sparrow". This takes place at the end of congress.

Sutra 23 When a woman acts the part of a man, she has the following things to do in addition to the nine given above: the "pair of tongs", the "top", the "swing".

Sutra 24 When the woman holds the *lingam* in her *yoni*, draws it in, presses it, and keeps it thus in her for a long time, it is called the "pair of tongs".

Sutra 25 When, while engaged in congress, she turns round like a wheel, it is called the "top". This is learned by practice only.

Sura 26–27 When, on such an occasion, the man lifts up the middle part of his body, and the woman turns round her middle part, it is called the "swing".

Sutra 28 When the woman is tired, she should place her forehead on that of her lover, and should thus take rest without disturbing the union of the organs.

Sutra 29 And when the woman has rested herself the man should turn round and recommence the congress.

Sutra 30 There are also some verses on the subject as follows:
"Though a woman is reserved, and keeps her feelings concealed; yet when she gets on the top of a man, she then shows all her love and desire."

Sutra 31 "A man should gather from the actions of the woman of what disposition she is, and in what way she likes to be enjoyed."

Sutra 32 "A woman during her monthly courses, a woman who has given birth lately, a woman who is pregnant, and a woman who is fat should not be made to act the part of a man."

Chapter IX The *auparishtaka*, or mouth congress

Sutra 1 There are two kinds of eunuchs, those that are disguised as males and those that are disguised as females.

Sutras 2–4 Eunuchs disguised as females imitate their dress, speech, gestures, tenderness, timidity, simplicity, softness and bashfulness. The acts that are done on the *jaghana* or middle parts of women, are done in the mouths of these eunuchs, and this is called *auparishtaka*.[11] These eunuchs derive their imaginable pleasure, and their livelihood, from this kind of congress, and they lead the life of courtesans.

Sutra 5 Eunuchs disguised as males keep their desires secret, and when they wish to do anything they lead the life of shampooers.

Sutra 6 Under the pretence of shampooing, a eunuch of this kind embraces and draws toward himself the thighs of the man whom he is shampooing, and after this he touches the joints of his thighs and his *jaghana*, or central portions of his body.

Sutra 7 Then, if he finds the *lingam* of the man erect, he presses it with his hands and chafes him for getting into that state.

Sutra 8 If after this, and after knowing his intention, the man does not tell the eunuch to proceed, then the latter does it of his own accord and begins the congress. If however he is ordered by the man to do it, then he disputes with him, and only consents at last with difficulty.

Sutra 9–11 The following eight things are then done by the eunuch one after the other: the "nominal congress", "biting the sides", "pressing outside", "pressing inside", "kissing", "rubbing", "sucking a mango fruit", "swallowing up".

At the end of each of these, the eunuch expresses his wish to stop, but when one of them is finished, the man desires him to do another, and after that is done, then the one that follows it, and so on.

Sutra 12 When, holding the man's *lingam* with his hand, and placing it between his lips, the eunuch moves about his mouth, it is called the "nominal congress".

Sutra 13 When, covering the end of the *lingam* with his fingers collected together like the bud of a plant or flower, the eunuch presses the sides of it with his lips, using his teeth also, it is called "biting the sides".

Sutra 14 When, being desired to proceed, the eunuch presses the end of the *lingam* with his lips closed together and kisses it as if he were drawing it out, it is called the "outside pressing".

Sutra 15 When, being asked to go on, he puts the *lingam* further into his mouth, presses it with his lips and then takes it out, it is called the "inside pressing".

Sutra 16 When, holding the *lingam* in his hand, the eunuch kisses it as if he were kissing the lower lip, it is called "kissing".

Sutra 17 When, after kissing it, he touches it with his tongue everywhere and passes the tongue over the end of it, it is called "rubbing".

Sutra 18 When, in the same way, he puts half of it into his mouth and forcibly kisses and sucks it, this is called "sucking a mango fruit".

Sutra 19 And lastly, when, with the consent of the man, the eunuch puts the whole *lingam* into his mouth, and presses it to the very end, as if he were going to swallow it up, it is called "swallowing up".

Sutra 20 Striking, scratching, and other things may also be done during this kind of congress.

Sutra 21 The *auparishtaka* is practised also by unchaste and wanton women, female attendants and serving maids; that is, those who are not married to anybody, but who live by shampooing.

Sutra 22 The *acharya*s (that is, ancient and venerable authors) are of the opinion that this *auparishtaka* is the work of a dog and not of a man, because it is a low practice, is contrary to the orders of the Holy Writ, and because the man himself suffers by bringing his *lingam* into contact with the mouths of eunuchs and women.

Sutra 23 But Vatsyayana says that the orders of the Holy Writ do not affect those who resort to courtesans, and the law prohibits the practice of the *auparishtaka* with married women only. As regards the injury to the male, that can be easily remedied.

Sutra 24 The people of eastern India do not resort to women who practise the *auparishtaka*. (They do unite with other types of women with whom they do not find fault.)

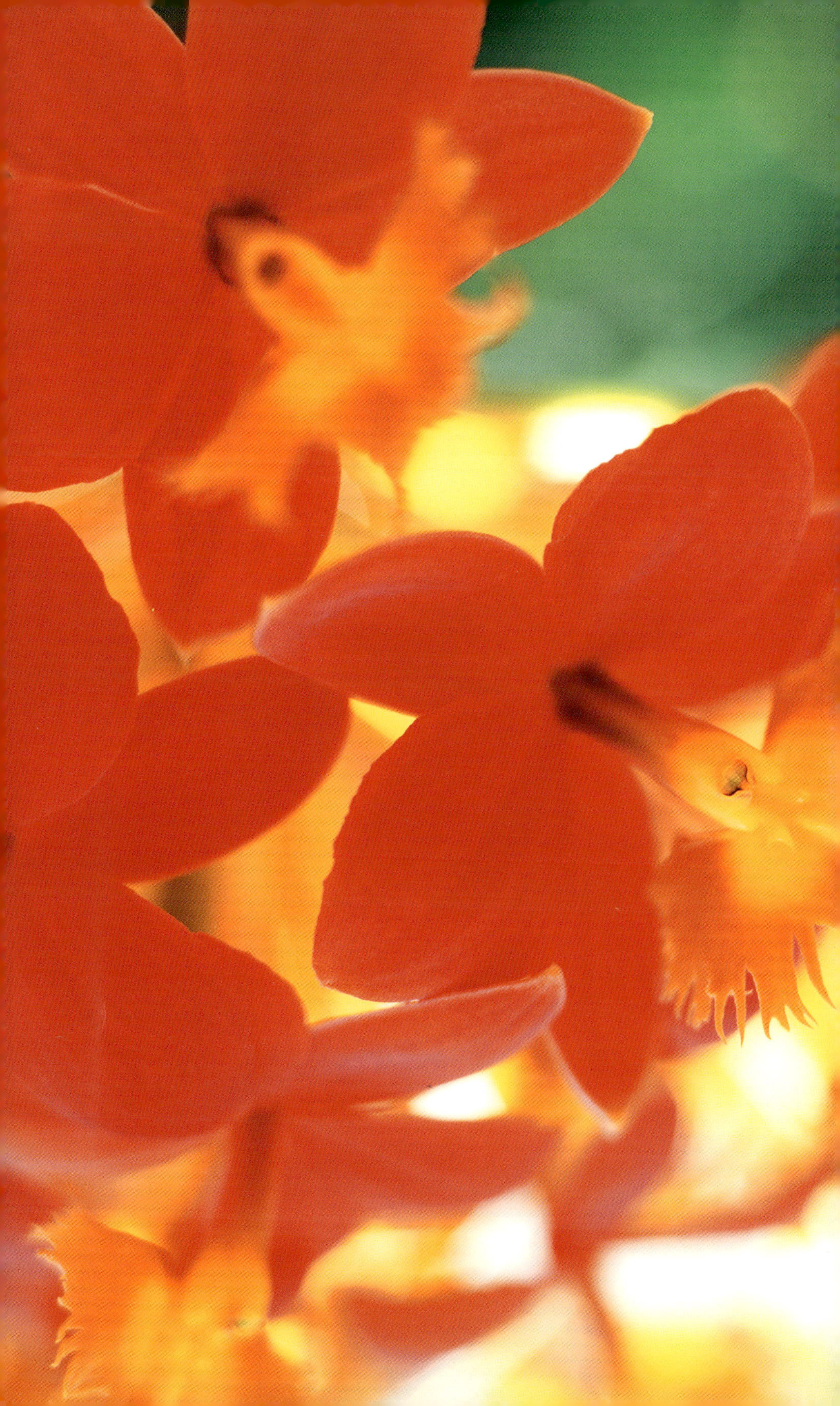

Sutra 25 The people of Ahichhatra resort to such women, but do nothing with them, so far as the mouth is concerned.

Sutra 26 The people of Saketa do every kind of mouth congress with these women, while the people of Nagara do not practise this, but do every other thing.

Sutras 27–29 The people of the Shurasena country, on the southern bank of the Jumna, do everything without any hesitation, for they say that because women are naturally unclean, no one can be certain about their character, their purity, their conduct, their practices, their confidences, or their speech.

They are not, however, to be abandoned on this account, because religious law, on the authority of which they are reckoned pure, lays down that the udder of a cow is clean at the time of milking, though the mouth of a cow and that of her calf are considered unclean. Again a dog is clean when he seizes a deer in hunting, though food touched by a dog is otherwise considered very unclean. A bird is clean when it causes a fruit to fall from a tree by pecking at it, though things eaten by crows and other birds are considered to be unclean. And the mouth of a woman is clean for kissing and such things at the time of sexual intercourse.

Sutra 30 Vatsyayana, moreover, thinks that in all these things connected with love, everybody should act according to the custom of his country, and his own inclination.

Sutra 31 There are also the following verses on the subject:

"The male servants of some men carry out mouth congress with their masters."

Sutra 32 "It is also practised by some citizens who know each other well, among themselves."

Sutra 33 "Some women of the harem, when they are amorous, do the acts of the mouth on the *yoni*s of one another, and some men do the same thing with women. The way of doing this (that is, of kissing the *yoni*) should be known from kissing the mouth."

Sutra 34 "When a man and woman lie down in an inverted order, with the head of the one toward the feet of the other, and conduct this congress, it is called the 'congress of a crow'."

Sutra 35 "For the sake of such things courtesans abandon men possessed of good qualities, liberal and clever, and become attached to low persons, such as slaves and elephant drivers."

Sutra 36 "The *auparishtaka*, or mouth congress, should never be indulged in by a Brahmin learned in sacred books, by a state official, or by a man of good reputation."

Sutra 37 "Although the practice is allowed by the *shastra*s, that is no reason to continue it, and then it need only be done in particular cases."

Sutra 38 "For example, the taste, the strength and the digestive qualities of dog meat are mentioned in works on medicine, but it does not follow that it should be eaten by the wise."

Sutra 39 "In the same way, there are some men, some places and some times, with respect to which use can be made of these practices."

Sutra 40 "A man should therefore pay regard to the place, the time and

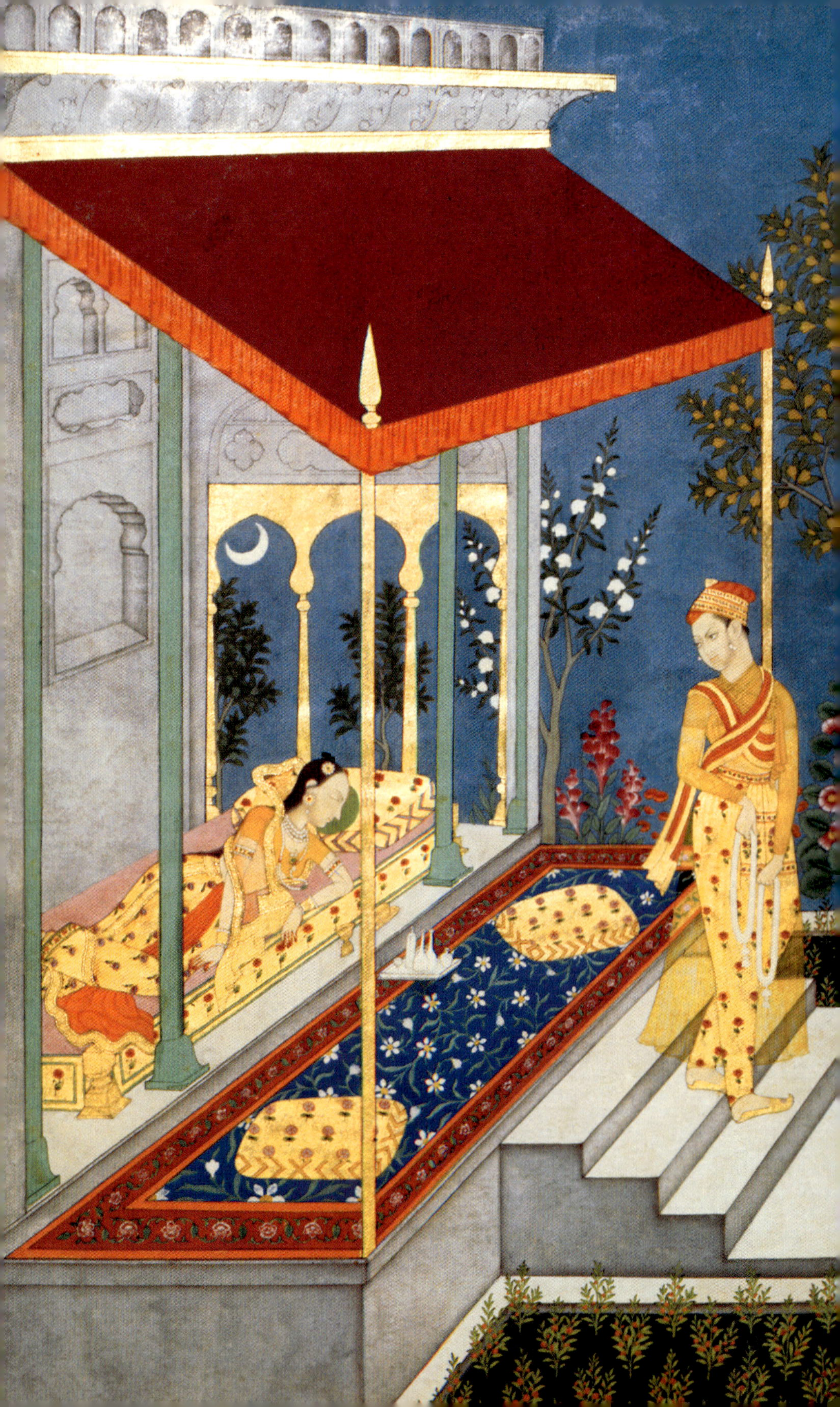

the practice which is to be carried out; also whether it is agreeable to his nature and to himself – and then he may or may not practise these things according to circumstances."

Sutra 41 "But after all, these things being done secretly and the mind of the man being fickle, how can it be known what any person will do at any particular time and for any particular purpose."

Chapter X The way to begin and to end the congress

Different kinds of congress and love quarrels

Sutras 1–12 In the pleasure-room, decorated with flowers and fragrant with perfumes, attended by his friends and servants, the citizen should receive the woman, who will come bathed and dressed, and will invite her to take refreshment and to drink freely. He should then seat her on his left side, and holding her hair, and touching also the end and knot of her garment, he should gently embrace her with his right arm. They should then carry on an amusing conversation on various subjects, and may also talk suggestively of things which would be considered as coarse, or not to be mentioned generally in society. They may then sing, either with or without gesticulations, and play on musical instruments, talk about the arts, and persuade each other to drink. At last, when the woman is overcome with love and desire, the citizen should dismiss the people that may be with him, giving them flowers, ointments and betel leaves, and then when the two are left alone, they should proceed as has been already described in the previous chapters.

Sutras 13–22 Such is the beginning of sexual union. At the end of the congress, the lovers, with modesty and not looking at each other, should go separately to the washing-room. After this, sitting in their own places, they should eat some betel leaves, and the citizen should apply with his own hand to the body of the woman some pure sandalwood ointment, or ointment of some other kind. He should then embrace her with his left arm, and with agreeable words should cause her to drink from a cup held in his own hand, or he may give her water to drink. They can then eat sweetmeats, or anything else, according to their likings and may drink fresh juice, soup, gruel, extracts of meat, sherbet, the juice of mango fruits, the extract of the juice of the citron tree mixed with sugar, or anything that may be liked in different countries and known to be sweet, soft and pure. The lovers may also sit on the terrace of the palace or house, enjoy the moonlight and carry on an agreeable conversation. At this time, too, while the woman lies in his lap, with her face toward the moon, the citizen should show her the different planets, the morning star, the polar star, and the seven *rishis*, or Great Bear.

This is the end of sexual union.

Sutras 23–27 Lovers will find that if they take their time in pleasing one another and foster confidence in one another, both at the commencent and conclusion of congress, the love between them will be heightened.

Sutra 28 Congress is of the following kinds: "loving congress", "congress of subsequent love", "congress of artificial love", "congress of transferred love", "congress like that of eunuchs", "deceitful congress" and "congress of spontaneous love".

Sutra 29 When a man and a woman, who have been in love with each other for some time, come together with great difficulty, or when one of the two returns from a journey, or is reconciled after having been separated on account of a quarrel, then their congress is called the "loving congress".

Sutra 30 The congress is carried on according to the liking of the lovers, and for as long as they choose.

Sutra 31 When two persons come together while their love for each other is still in its infancy, their congress is called the "congress of subsequent love".

Sutras 32–33 When a man carries on the congress by exciting himself by means of the sixty-four ways, such as kissing, and so on, or when a man and a woman come together, though in reality they are both attached to different persons, their congress is then called "congress of artificial love". At this time all the ways and means mentioned in the *Kama Shastra* should be used.

Sutra 34 When a man, from the beginning to the end of the congress, though having connection with the woman, thinks all the time that he is enjoying another one whom he loves, it is called the "congress of transferred love".

Sutras 35–36 Congress between a man and a female water carrier, or a female servant of a caste lower than his own, lasting only until the desire is satisfied, is called "congress like that of eunuchs". Here external touches, kisses and manipulation are not to be employed.

Sutras 37–38 The congress between a courtesan and a rustic, and that between citizens and the women of villages and bordering countries, is called "deceitful congress".

Sutra 39 The congress that takes place between two persons who are attached to one another, and which is done according to their own liking, is called "congress of spontaneous love".

Thus end the kinds of congress.

Sutra 40 We shall now speak of love quarrels.

A woman who is very much in love with a man cannot bear to hear the name of her rival in love mentioned, or to have any conversation regarding her, or to hear her being praised, or to be addressed by him using her rival's name by mistake.

Sutra 41 If such takes place, a great quarrel arises and the woman cries, becomes angry, tosses her hair about, strikes her lover, falls from her bed or seat, and, casting aside her garlands and ornaments, throws herself down on the ground.

Sutra 42 At this time, the lover should remain unperturbed, try to placate her with conciliatory words, and should take her up and place her on her bed.

Sutras 43–44 But she, not replying to his questions, and with increased anger, should bend down his head by pulling his hair, and having kicked him once, twice or thrice on his arms, head, bosom or back, should then proceed to the door of the room.

Sutra 45 Dattaka says that she should then sit angrily near the door and shed tears, but should not go out, because she would be found fault with for going away.

Sutra 46 After a time, when she thinks that the conciliatory words and actions of her lover have reached their utmost, she should then embrace him, talking to him with harsh and reproachful words, but at the same time showing a loving desire for congress.

Sutra 47 When the woman is in her own house, and has quarrelled with her lover, she should go to him and show how angry she is, and leave him.

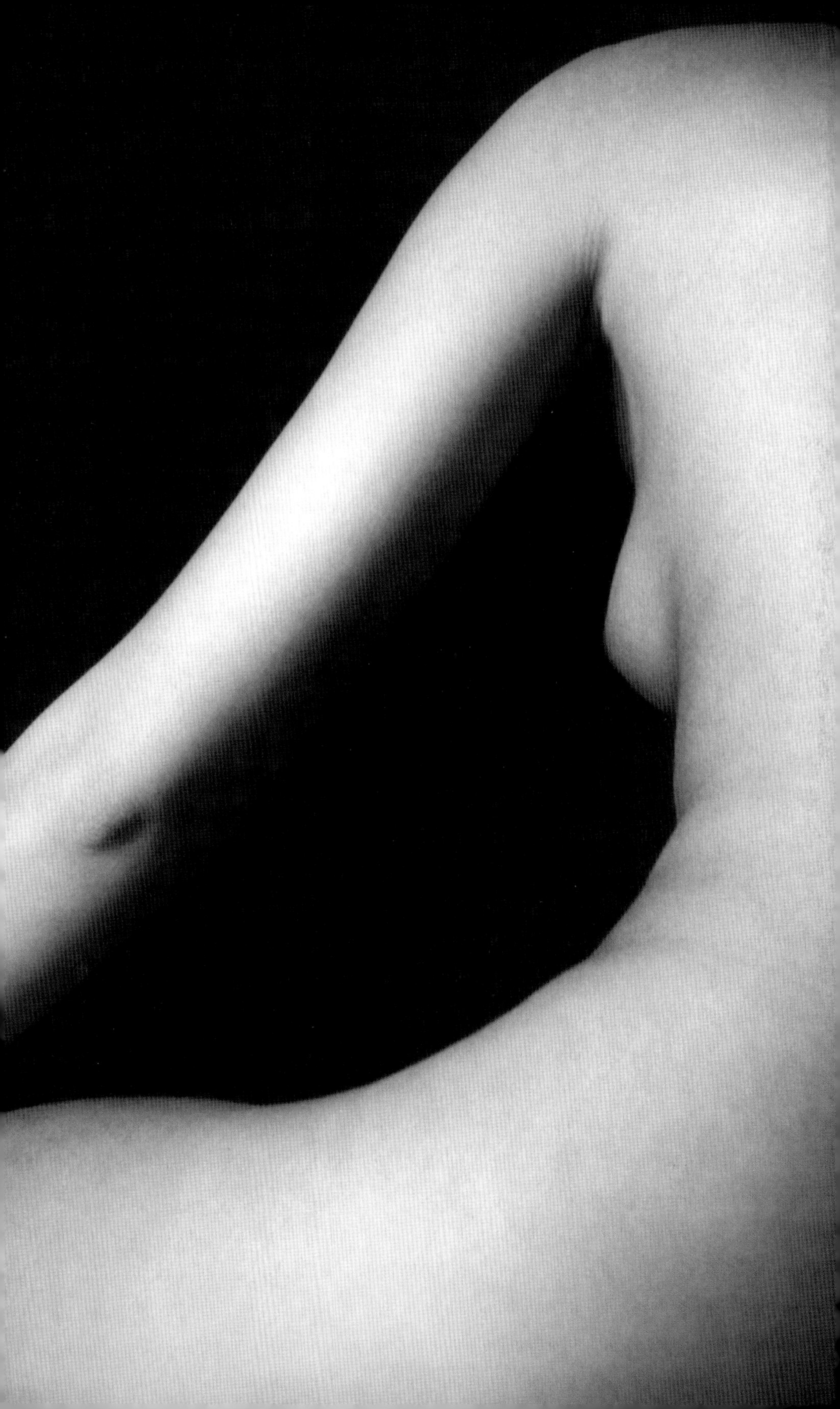

Sutra 48 Afterwards, the citizen having sent the *vita*, the *vidushaka* or the *pithamarda*[12] to pacify her, she should accompany them back to the house and spend the night with her lover.

Thus ends consideration of love quarrels.

Sutra 49 In conclusion.

A man who is well versed in the sixty-four arts mentioned by Babhravya can succeed in his objective and win over women of the highest quality.

Sutra 50 Although he may speak well on other subjects, if he does not know the sixty-four arts no great respect is paid to him in the assembly of the learned.

Sutra 51 A man, devoid of other knowledge, but well acquainted with the sixty-four arts, becomes a leader in any society of men and women.

Sutra 52 What man will not respect the sixty-four arts[13] given that they are respected by the learned, by the cunning and by the courtesans?

Sutras 53–54 As the sixty-four arts are respected, are charming, and add to the talent of women, they are deemed dear to women by the *acharyas*. A man skilled in the sixty-four arts is looked upon with love by his own wife, by the wives of others and by courtesans.

NOTES

1. *Lingam* connotes the penis.
2. *Yoni* connotes the vagina.
3. In high unions it is possible for men to satisfy their own passion without injuring the female, while in low unions it is difficult for the female to be satisfied by any means.
4. The strength of passion within women varies a great deal, some being easily satisfied and others eager and willing to go on for a long time. To satisfy these last thoroughly a man must have recourse to art. It is certain that a fluid flows from the woman in larger or smaller quantities, but her satisfaction is not complete until she has experienced the "*spasme*" *génital*, as described in a French work recently published called *Breviare de l'Amour Expérimental.*
5. This is a long dissertation very common among Sanskrit authors.
6. In actual fact the number is 729.
7. This paragraph should be particularly noted, for it specially applies to married men and their wives. So many men utterly ignore the feelings of the women, and never pay the slightest attention to the passion of the latter. To understand the subject thoroughly, it is absolutely necessary to study it, and then a person will know that, as dough is prepared for baking, so must a woman be prepared for sexual intercourse, if she is to derive satisfaction from it.
8. From this it would appear that in ancient times the breasts of women were not covered, and this is seen in the paintings of the Ajunta and other caves, where we find that the breasts of even royal ladies and others are exposed.
9. Medicine being a reference to the use of "mechanical aids".
10. Men who are well acquainted with the art of love are well aware how often one woman differs from another in her sighs and sounds during the time of congress. Some women like to be talked to in the most loving way, others in the most lustful way, others in the most abusive way, and so on. Some women enjoy themselves with closed eyes in silence, others make a great noise of it, and some almost faint away. The great art is to ascertain what gives them the greatest pleasure, and what specialities they like best.
11. This practice appears to have been prevalent in some parts of India from a very ancient time. The *Shustruta*, a work on medicine some 2,000 years old, describes the wounding of the *lingam* with the teeth as one of the causes of a disease, treatment for which is described in that work. Traces of the practice are found as far back as the eighth century, for various kinds of the *auparishtaka* are represented in the sculptures of many temples at Bhubaneshwar, in Orissa, which were built about that period. These sculptures suggest that the practice was popular in that part of the country at that time. It does not seem to be so prevalent now.
12. See page 43, notes 13, 17, 19 and 20.
13. See pages 25–28.

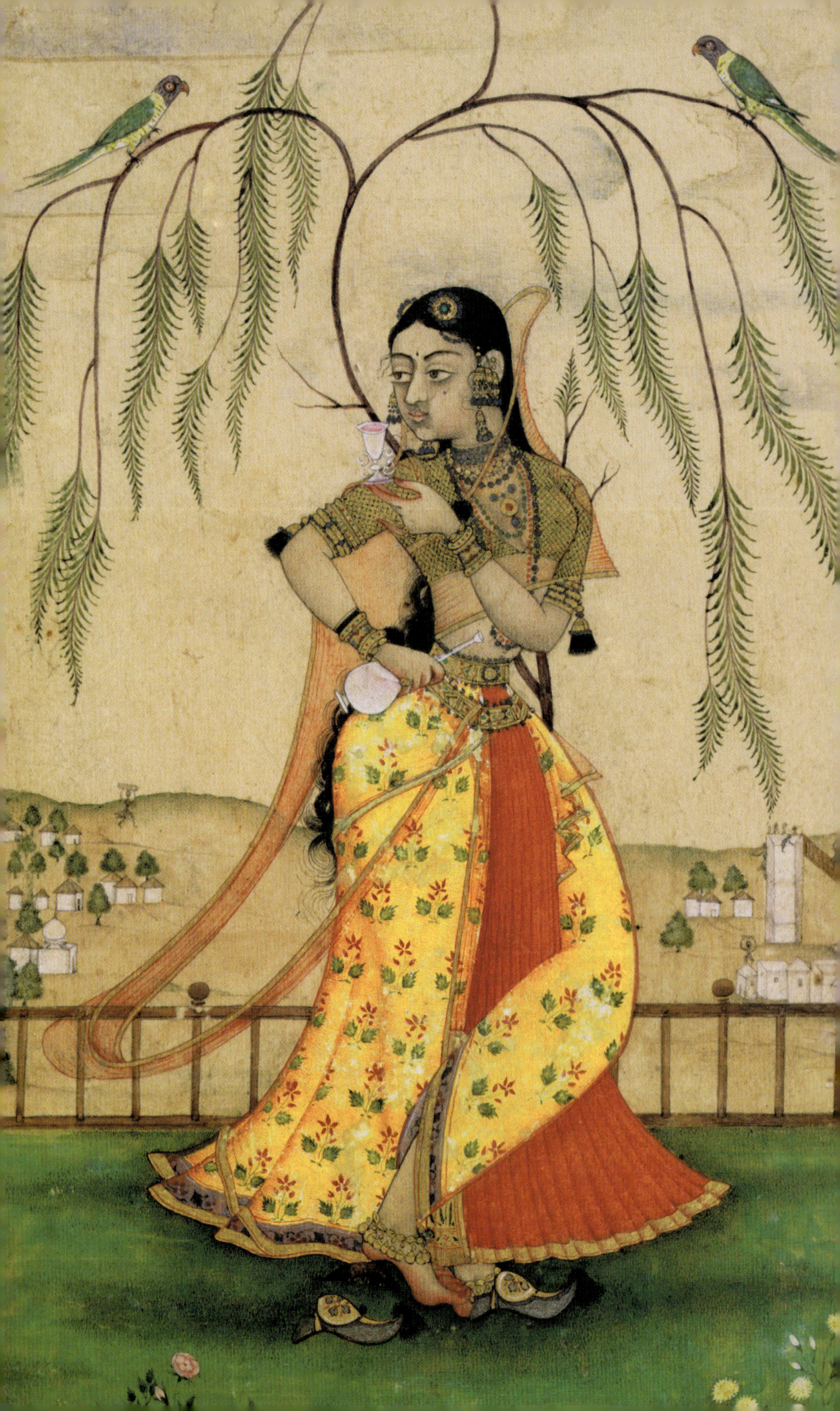

Part Three: On Acquiring a Wife

Chapter I On marriage

Sutra 1 When a girl of the same caste, and a virgin, is married in accordance with the precepts of Holy Writ, the results of such a union are the acquisition of Dharma and Artha, offspring, affinity, more friends and untarnished love.

Sutra 2 For this reason a man should fix his affections upon a girl who is of good family, whose parents are alive, and who is three years or more younger than himself. She should be born of a highly respectable family, possessed of wealth, well connected, and with many relations and friends. She should also be beautiful, of a good disposition, with lucky marks on her body, and with good hair, nails, teeth, ears, eyes and breasts, neither more nor less than they ought to be, and no one of them entirely wanting, and not troubled with a sickly body. The man must, of course, also possess the same qualities he expects in his bride.

Sutra 3 But at all events, says Ghotakamukha, a girl who has already been joined with others (that is, no longer a maiden) should never be loved, for it would be reproachable to do such a thing.

Sutra 4 Now in order to bring about a marriage with such a girl as described above, the parents and relations of the man should exert themselves, as also should friends of the two sides.

Sutras 5–6 These friends should bring to the notice of the girl's parents, the faults, both present and future, of all the other men that may wish to marry her, and should at the same time extol – even exaggerate – all the excellencies, ancestral and paternal, of their friend, so as to endear him to them, and particularly those that may be liked by the girl's mother.

Sutras 7–8 One of the friends should also disguise himself as an astrologer, and declare the future good fortune and wealth of his friend by showing the existence of all the lucky omens[1] and signs,[2] the good influence of planets, the auspicious entrance of the sun into a sign of the zodiac, propitious stars and fortunate marks on his body.

The astrologer may rouse the jealousy of the girl's mother by telling her that the friend has a chance of getting from some other quarter an even better girl than hers.

Sutras 9–10 A girl should be taken as a wife, and given in marriage, when fortune, signs, omens and the words[3] of others are favourable, for, says Ghotakamukha, a man should not marry at any time he likes.

Sutra 11 A girl who is asleep, crying or out of the house when sought in marriage, or who is betrothed to another, should not be married.

Sutra 12 The following should also be avoided:

One who is kept concealed

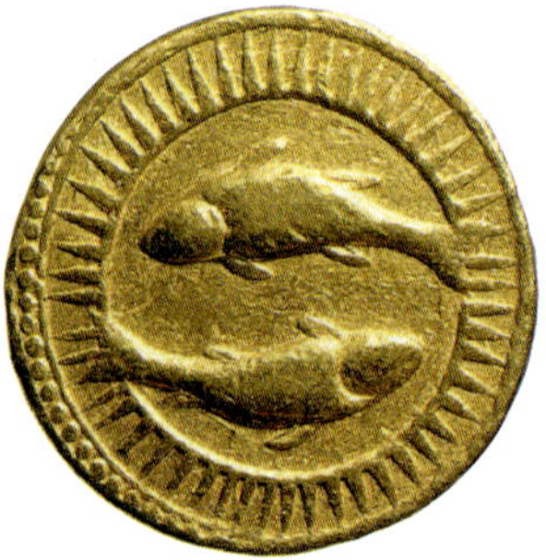

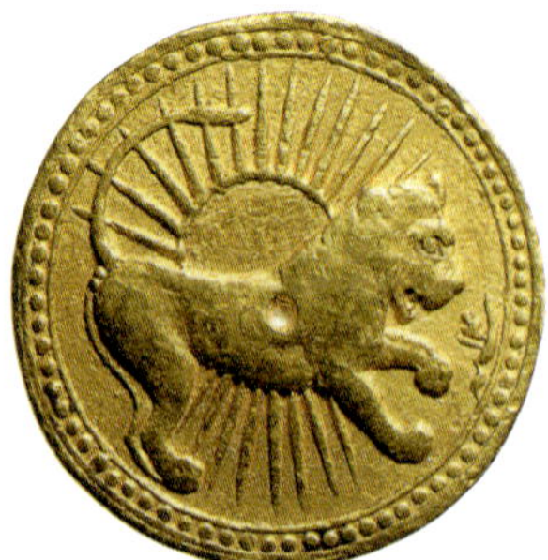

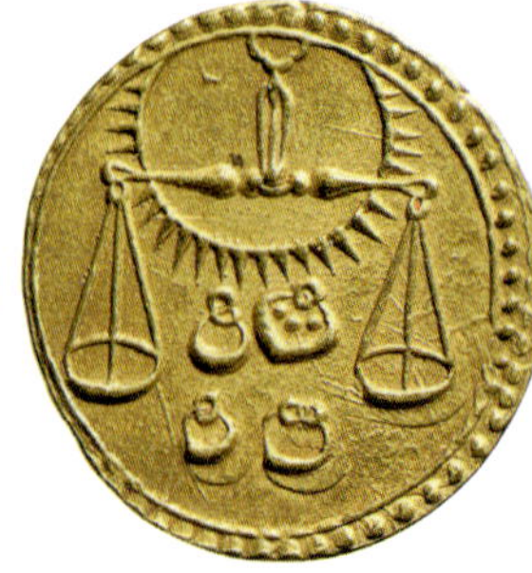

One who has an inauspicious name
One who has her nose depressed
One who has her nostril turned up
One who is built like a male
One who is stooped
One who has crooked thighs
One who has a prominent forehead
One who has a bald head
One who does not like purity
One who has been polluted by another
One who is affected with the *gulma*[4]
One who is disfigured in any way
One who has fully arrived at puberty
One who is a friend
One who is a younger sister

Sutra 13 In the same way a girl who bears the name of one of twenty-seven stars, a tree or a river is considered worthless, as too is a girl whose name ends in "r" or "l".

Sutra 14 But some sages say that prosperity is gained only by marrying that girl to whom one becomes attached, and that therefore no other girl but the one who is loved should be married by anyone.

Sutra 15 When a girl becomes marriageable her parents should dress her smartly, and should place her where she can be seen easily by all.

Sutra 16 Every afternoon, having dressed her and decorated her in a becoming manner, they should send her with her female companions to sports, sacrifices and marriage ceremonies, and thus show her to advantage in society, because she is a kind of merchandise.

Sutras 17–18 They should also receive with kind words and signs of friendliness those of an auspicious appearance who may come accompanied by their friends and relations for the purpose of marrying their daughter, and under some pretext or other – having first dressed her becomingly – they should then present her to them.

Sutra 19 After this they should await the pleasure of fortune, and with this object should appoint a future day on which a determination could be reached with regard to their daughter's marriage.

Sutra 20 On this occasion, when the persons have come, the parents of the girl should ask them to bathe and dine, and should say, "Everything will take place at the proper time", and should not then comply with the request, but should settle the matter later.

Sutra 21 When a marriage has been arranged, the man should wed the girl in accordance with the precepts of the Holy Writ, according to one of the four kinds of marriage. Thus ends consideration of marriage.

Sutras 22–26 There are also some verses on the subject as follows: "Amusement in society, such as completing verses begun by others, marriages and auspicious ceremonies should be carried on neither with superiors, nor inferiors, but with our equals. That should be known as a high connection when a man, after marrying a girl, has to serve her and her relations afterwards like a servant, and such a connection is censured by the good. On the other hand, that reproachable connection, where a man, together with his relations, lords it over his wife, is called a low connection by the wise. But when both the man and the woman afford mutual pleasure to each other, and when the relatives on both sides pay respect to one another, such is called a connection in the proper sense of the word. Therefore a man should contract neither a high connection,

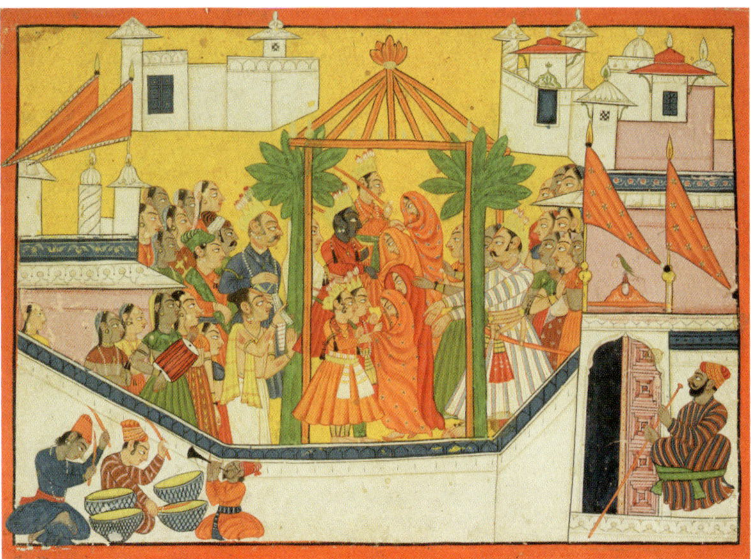

by which he is obliged to bow down afterwards to his kinsmen, nor a low connection, which is universally reprehended by all."

Chapter II Creating confidence in the girl

Sutra 1 For the first three days after marriage, the girl and her husband should sleep on the floor, abstain from sexual pleasures, and eat their food without seasoning it either with alkali or salt. For the next seven days they should bathe accompanied by the sounds of auspicious musical instruments, should decorate themselves, dine together, and pay attention to their relations as well as to those who may have come to witness their marriage. This is applicable to persons of all four castes.

Sutra 2 On the night of the tenth day the man should begin in a secluded place with soft words, and thus create confidence in the girl.

Sutra 3 Some authors say that for the purpose of winning her over he should not speak to her for three days, but the followers of Babhravya are of opinion that if the man does not speak with the girl for three days she may be discouraged by seeing him spiritless like a pillar, and, becoming dejected, may begin to despise him as a eunuch.

Sutra 4 Vatsyayana says that the man should begin to win her over, and to create confidence in her, but should abstain at first from sexual pleasures.

Sutras 5–6 Women, being of a tender nature, want tender beginnings, and when they are forcibly approached by men with whom they are but slightly acquainted, they sometimes suddenly become haters of sexual connection, and sometimes even haters of the male sex. The man should therefore approach the girl according to her liking, and should make use of those devices by which he may be able to establish himself more and more into her confidence.

Sutra 7 These devices are as follows:

Sutras 8–9 He should embrace her first of all in a way she likes most, because it does not last for a long time.

Sutra 10 He should embrace her with the upper part of his body because that is easier and simpler. If the girl is grown up, or if the man has known her for some time, he may embrace her by the light of a lamp, but if he is not well acquainted with her, or if she is a young girl, he should then embrace her in darkness.

Sutra 11 When the girl accepts the embrace, the man should put a *tambula* or screw of betel nut and betel leaves in her mouth, and if she will not take it, he should induce her to do so by conciliatory words, entreaties, oaths and kneeling at her feet, for it is a universal rule that however bashful or angry a woman may be she never disregards a man's kneeling at her feet.

Sutra 12 At the time of giving this *tambula* he should kiss her mouth softly and gracefully without making any sound.

Sutras 13–14 When she is gained over in this respect he should then make her talk, and so that she may be induced to talk he should ask her questions about things of which he knows or pretends to know nothing, and which can be answered in a few words.

Sutra 15 If she does not speak to him, he should not frighten her, but should ask her the same thing again and again in a conciliatory manner.

Sutras 16–17 If she does not then speak he should urge her to give a reply, because as Ghotakamukha says, "All girls hear everything said to them by men, but do not themselves sometimes say a single word".

Sutra 18 When she is thus importuned, the girl should reply by shakes of the head, but if she has quarrelled with the man she should not even do that.

Sutra 19 When she is asked by the man whether she wishes for him, and whether she likes him, she should remain silent for a long time, and when at last importuned to reply, should give him a favourable answer by a nod of her head.

Sutra 20 If the man is previously acquainted with the girl he should converse through a female friend, who may be favourable to him and in the confidence of both, and carry on the conversation on both sides.

Sutra 21 In such circumstances the girl should smile with her head bent down during the conversation.

Sutra 22 Then, if the female friend says more on her part than it was desired, she should rebuke her.

Sutras 23–26 The female friend should say in jest what she is not desired to say by the girl, and add, "she says so", upon which the girl should say indistinctly and prettily, "Oh no! I did not say so", and she should then smile and throw an occasional glance toward the man.

Sutra 27 If the girl is familiar with the man, she should place near him, without saying anything, the *tambula*, the ointment, or the garland that he may have asked for, or she may tie them up in his upper garment.

Sutra 28 While she is engaged in this, the man should touch her young breasts in the "sounding" way of pressing with the nails. [See page 64.]

Sutra 29 And if she prevents him doing this he should say to her, "I will not do it again if you will embrace me", and should in this way cause her to embrace him. While he is being embraced by her he should pass his hand repeatedly over and about her body. By and by he should place her in his lap, and try more and more to gain her consent.

Sutra 30 And if she will not respond to him he should frighten her by saying, "I shall impress marks of my teeth and nails on your lips and breasts, and then make similar marks on my own body, and shall tell my friends that you did them. What will you say then?" In this and other ways, not unlike resorting to the tricks used to frighten children into acquiescence, so should the man be able to win her over gradually to his wishes.

Sutra 31 On the second and third nights, after her confidence has increased more, he should feel the whole of her body with his hands.

Sutras 32–33 He should now kiss her all over; he should also place his hands upon her thighs and shampoo them.

Sutras 34–35 And if he succeeds in this he should then shampoo the joints of her thighs. If she tries to prevent him doing this he should say to her, "What harm is there in doing it?" and should persuade her to let him do it. After gaining this point he should touch her private parts, should loosen her girdle and the knot of her dress, and turning up her lower garment should shampoo the joints of her naked thighs.

Sutra 36 Under various pretences he should do all these things, but he should not at that time begin actual congress.

Sutras 37–38 After this he should teach her the sixty-four arts, should tell her how much he loves her, and describe to her the hopes which he formerly entertained regarding her. He should also promise to be faithful to her in future, and should dispel all her fears with respect to rival women, and, at last, after having overcome her bashfulness, he should begin to enjoy her in a way so as not to frighten her.

So much about creating confidence in the girl.

Sutra 39 And there are, moreover, some verses on the subject as follows: "A man acting according to the inclinations of a girl should try to gain her over so that she may love him and place her confidence in him."

Sutra 40 "A man does not succeed either by implicitly following the inclination of a girl, or by wholly opposing her, and he should therefore adopt a middle course."

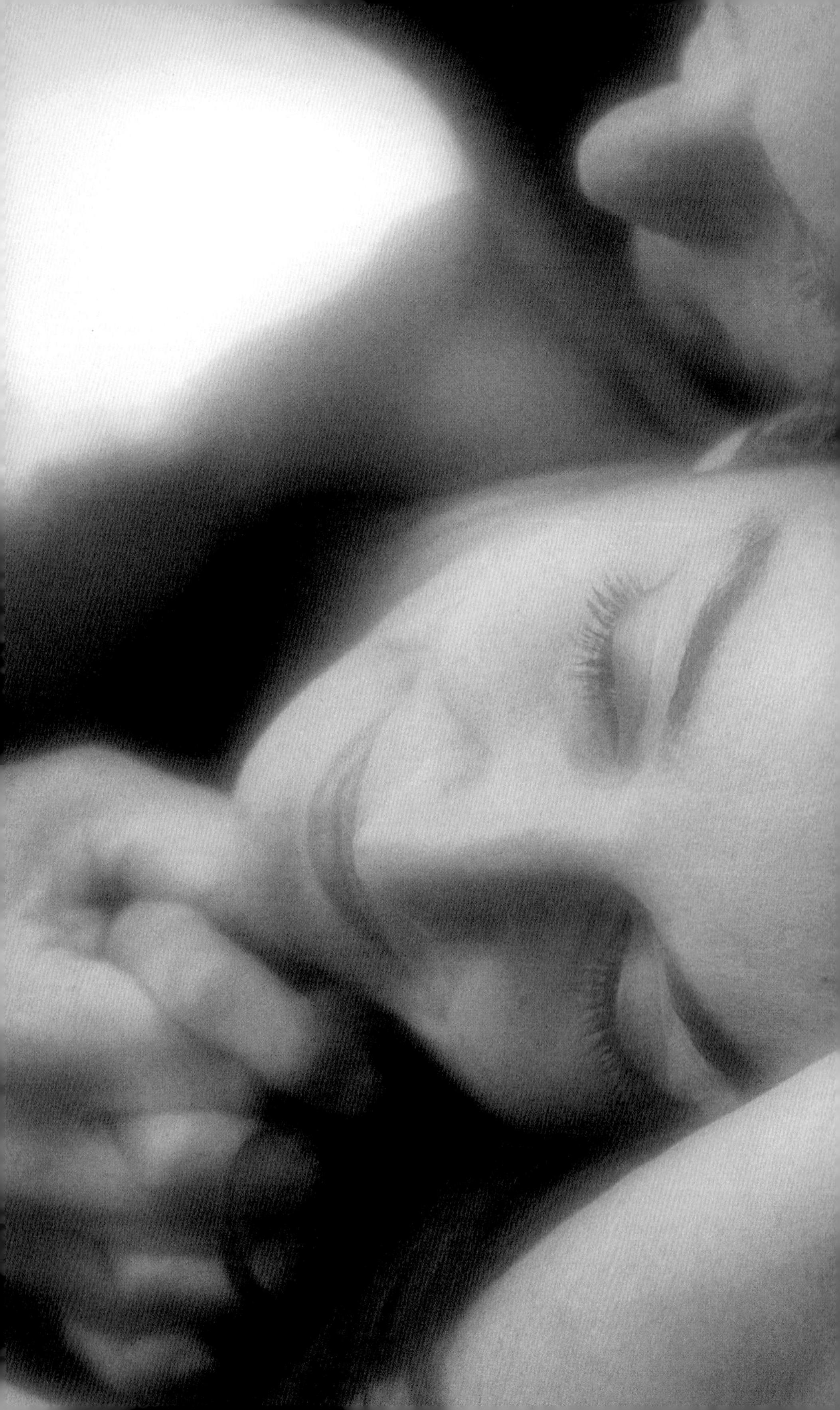

Sutra 41 "He who knows how to make himself beloved by women, as well as to increase their honour and create confidence in them, this man becomes an object of their love."

Sutra 42 "But he who neglects a girl, thinking she is too bashful, is despised by her as a beast ignorant of the working of the female mind."

Sutras 43–44 "Moreover, a girl forcibly enjoyed by one who does not understand the hearts of girls becomes nervous, uneasy and dejected, and suddenly begins to hate the man who has taken advantage of her; and then, when her love is not understood or returned, she sinks into despondency, and becomes either a hater of mankind altogether, or, hating her own man, she has recourse to other men."

Chapter III On courtship, and the manifestation of the feelings by outward signs and deeds

Sutras 1–2 A poor man, though he may be blessed with good qualities, or a man of low birth, though he may possess mediocre qualities, or a neighbour, though he may be wealthy, or one who has to depend on his father, mother or brothers for a livelihood, should not marry unless he has endeavoured to win over the girl to love and esteem him from as early as her childhood.

Sutra 3 Thus a boy orphaned from his parents, and living in the house of his uncle, should try to woo the daughter of his uncle even though she be previously betrothed to another.

Sutra 4 And this way of gaining over a girl, says Ghotakamukha, is unexceptional, because Dharma can be accomplished by means of it as well as by any other way of marriage.

Sutras 5–6 When a boy has thus begun to woo the girl he loves, he should spend his time with her and amuse her with various games and diversions fitted for their age and acquaintanceship, such as picking and collecting flowers, making garlands of flowers, playing the parts of members of a fictitious family, cooking food, playing with dice, playing with cards, the game of odd and even, the game of finding out the middle finger, the game of six pebbles, and such other games as may be prevalent in the country and agreeable to the disposition of the girl.

Sutra 7 In addition to this, he should carry on various amusing games played by several persons together, such as hide-and-seek, playing with seeds, hiding things in several small heaps of wheat and looking for them, blindman's buff, gymnastic exercises and other games of the same sort, in company with the girl, her friends and female attendants.

Sutra 8 The man should also show great kindness to any woman whom the girl thinks fit to be trusted, and should also make new acquaintances.

Sutra 9 But above all he should attach to himself by kindness and little services the daughter of the girl's nurse, for if she be gained over, even though she comes to know of his design, she does not cause any obstruction, but is sometimes even able to effect a union between him and the girl.

Sutra 10 And though she knows the true character of the man, she always talks of his many excellent qualities to the parents and relations of the girl, even though she may not be desired to do so by him.

Sutra 11–12 In this way the man should do whatever the girl takes most delight in, and he should get for her whatever she may have a

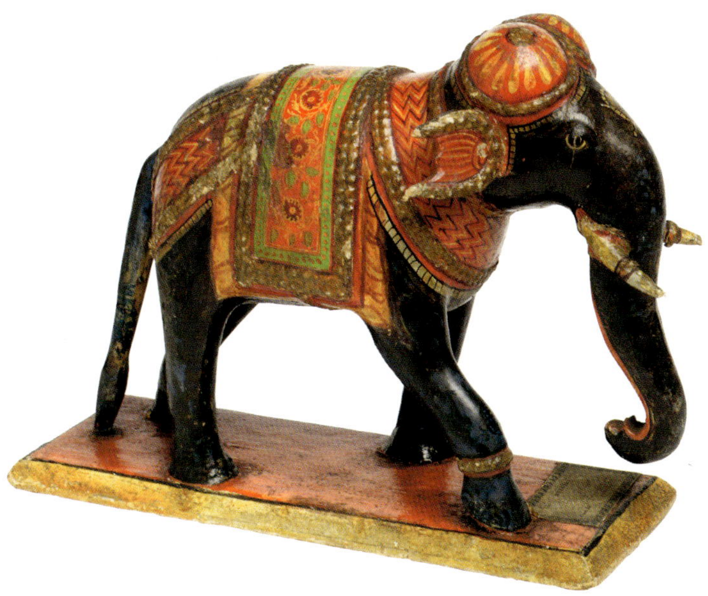

desire to possess. Thus he should procure for her such playthings as may be hardly known to other girls.

Sutra 13 He may also show her a ball dyed with various colours, and other curiosities of the same sort; and should give her dolls made of cloth, wood, buffalo-horn, wax, flour or clay.

Sutras 14–15 Also utensils for cooking food, and figures in wood, such as a man and woman standing, a pair of rams, goats or sheep; also temples made of clay, bamboo or wood, dedicated to various goddesses; and cages for parrots, cuckoos, starlings, quails, cocks and partridges; water-vessels of different sorts and of elegant forms, machines for throwing water about, guitars, stands for putting images upon, stools, lac, red arsenic, yellow ointment, vermilion and collyrium, as well as sandalwood, saffron, betel nut and betel leaves. Such things should be given at different times whenever he gets a good opportunity of meeting her, and some of them should be given in private, and some in public, according to circumstances. In short, he should try in every way to make her look upon him as one who would do for her everything that she wanted to be done.

Sutra 16 In the next place he should get her to meet him in some place privately, and should then tell her that the reason for his giving presents to her in secret was the fear that the parents of both of them might be displeased, and then he may add that the things which he had given her had been much desired by other people.

Sutra 17 When her love begins to show signs of increasing he should relate to her agreeable stories if she expresses a wish to hear such tales.

Sutra 18 Or if she takes delight in conjuring, he should amaze her by performing various tricks of jugglery; or if she feels a great curiosity to see a performance of the various arts, he should show his own skill in them. When she is delighted with singing he should entertain her with music, and on certain days – when going together to moonlight fairs and festivals, and at the time of her return after being absent from home – he should present her with bouquets of flowers, with chaplets for the head, and with ear ornaments and rings, for these are the proper occasions on which such things should be presented.

Sutra 19 He should also teach the daughter of the girl's nurse the sixty-four means of pleasure practised by men.

Sutra 20 Under this pretext he should also inform her of his great skill in the art of sexual enjoyment.

Sutra 21 All this time he should wear a fine dress, and make as good an appearance as possible.

Sutras 22–23 For young women love men who live with them, and who are handsome, good looking and well dressed. As for the sayings that though women may fall in love, they still make no effort themselves to win over the object of their affections, that is only a matter of idle talk.

Sutra 24 Now a girl always shows her love by outward signs and actions, such as the following:

Sutra 25 She never looks the man in the face, and becomes abashed when she is looked at by him.

Sutra 26 Under some pretext or other she shows her limbs to him.

Sutra 27 She looks secretly at him though he is away from her side.

Sutra 28 She hangs down her head when asked some question by him, and answers in indistinct words and unfinished sentences.

Sutra 29 She delights to be in his company for a long time.

Sutra 30 When she is at a distance from him she speaks to her attendants in a peculiar tone with the hope of attracting his attention toward her, because she does not wish to go from the place where he is.

Sutra 31 Under some pretext or other she makes him look at different things, narrates to him tales and stories very slowly so that she may continue conversing with him for a long time.

Sutra 32 She kisses and embraces before him a child sitting in her lap, and draws ornamental marks on the foreheads of her female servants.

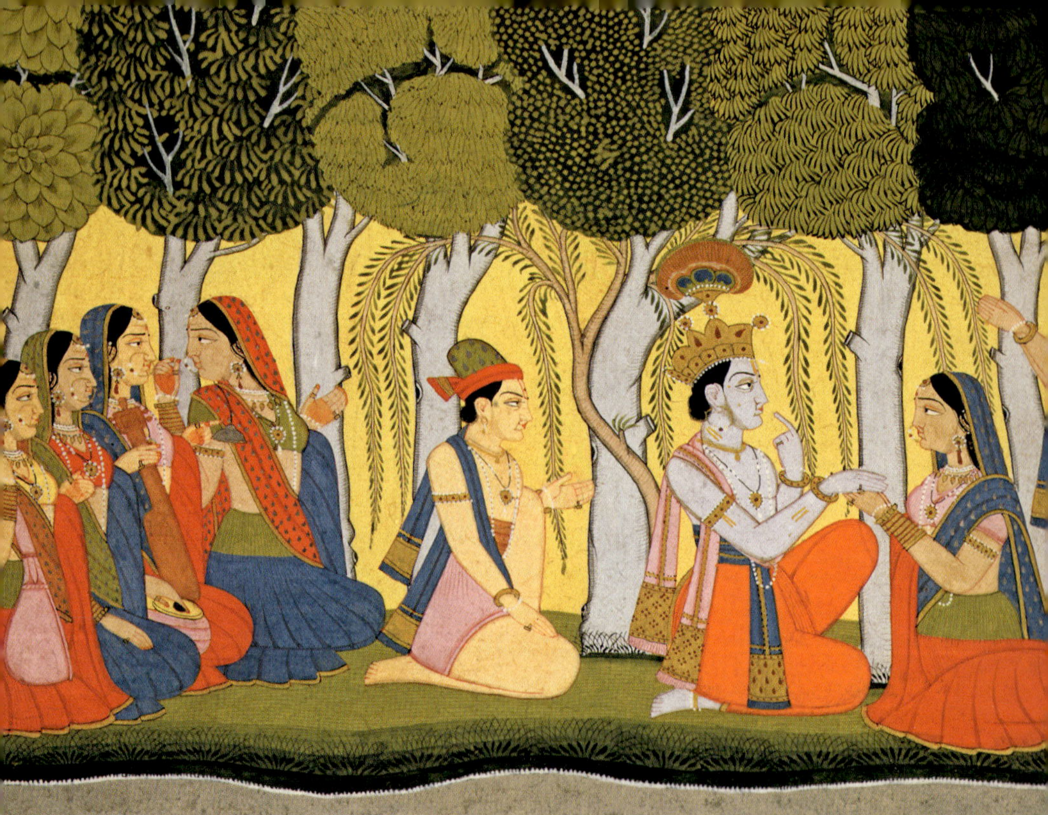

Sutra 33 She performs sportive and graceful movements when her attendants speak jestingly to her in the presence of her lover.

Sutra 34 She confides in her lover's friends, respecting them.

Sutra 35 She shows kindness to his servants and converses with them.

Sutra 36 She engages his servants to do her work as if she were their mistress.

Sutra 37 She listens attentively to his servants when they tell stories about her lover to somebody else.

Sutras 38–39 She enters his house when induced to do so by the daughter of her nurse, and by her assistance manages to converse and play with him.

Sutra 40 She avoids being seen by her lover when she is not dressed and decorated.

Sutra 41 She gives him – by the hand of her female friend – her ear ornament, ring or garland of flowers that he may have asked to see, and always wears anything that he may have presented to her.

Sutra 42 She becomes dejected when any other bridegroom is mentioned by her parents, and does not mix with those who may be of his party or who may support his claims.

Sura 43 There are also some verses on the subject as follows:
"A man, who has seen and perceived the feelings of the girl toward him, and who has noticed the outward signs and movements by which those feelings are expressed, should do everything in his power to effect a union with her."

Sutra 44 "He should gain over a young girl by childlike sports, a damsel come of age by his skill in the arts, and a girl that loves him by having recourse to persons in whom she confides."

Chapter IV Things to be done by the man to get the girl; and what is to be done by the girl to get the man and subject him to her

Sutra 1 Now when the girl begins to show her love by outward signs and motions, as described in the last chapter, the lover should try to gain her over entirely by various ways and means, such as the following:

Sutra 2 When engaged with her in any game or sport he should intentionally hold her hand.

Sutra 3 He should practise upon her the various kinds of embraces, such as the "touching embrace", and others already described in a preceding chapter. [See pages 52–57.]

Sutra 4–5 He should show her a pair of human beings cut out of the leaf of a tree, and such things, at intervals.

Sutra 6 When engaged in water sports, he should dive at a distance from her, and come up close to her.

Sutras 7–8 He should show an increased liking for the new foliage of trees and similar such things. He should describe to her the pangs he suffers on her account.

Sutra 9 He should relate to her the beautiful dream that he has had with reference to other women.

Sutras 10–15 At parties and assemblies of his caste he should sit near her, and touch her under some pretence or other, and having placed his foot upon hers, he should slowly touch each of her toes, and press the ends of the nails; if successful in this, he should get hold of her foot with his hand and repeat the same thing.

Sutra 16 He should also press a finger of her hand between his toes when she happens to be washing his feet.

Sutra 17 Whenever he gives anything to her or takes anything from her, he should show her by his manner and look how much he loves her.

Sutra 18 He should sprinkle upon her the water brought for rinsing his mouth.

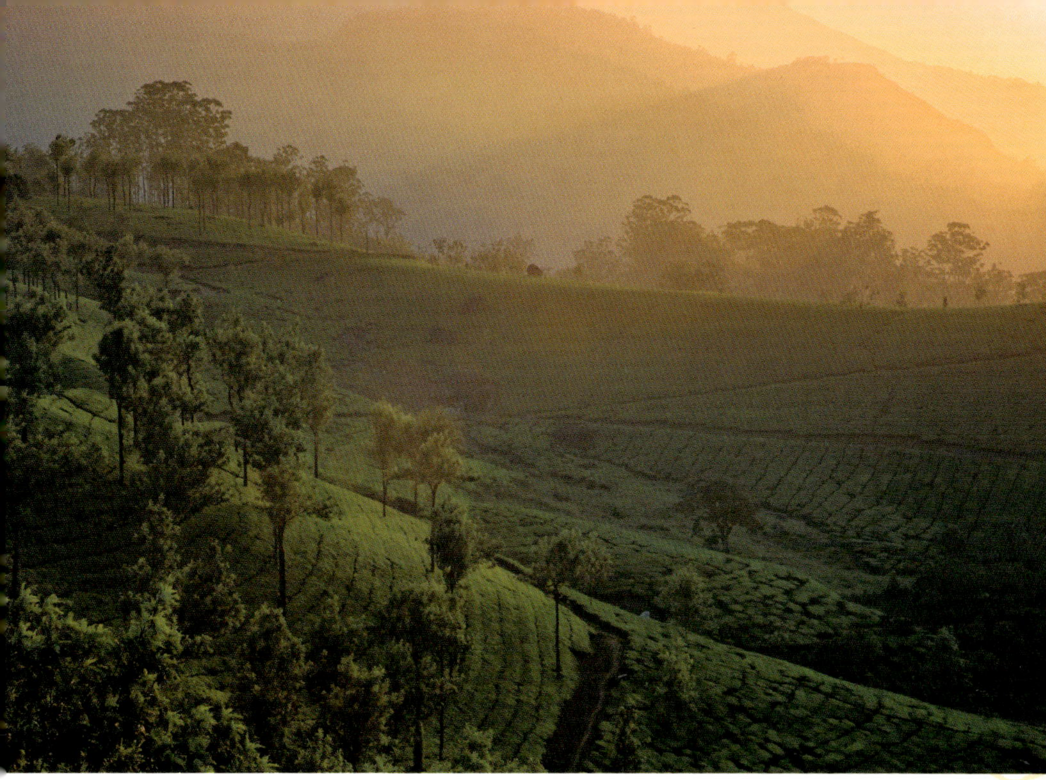

Sutra 19 And when alone with her in a secluded place, or in darkness, he should make love to her.

Sutra 20 And he should tell her the true state of his mind without distressing her in any way.

Sutra 21 Whenever he sits with her on the same seat or bed he should say to her, "I have something to tell you in private", and then, when she comes to hear it in a quiet place, he should express his love to her more by manner and signs than by words.

Sutra 22 When he comes to know the state of her feelings toward him he should pretend to be ill, and should make her come to his house to speak to him.

Sutra 23 There he should intentionally hold her hand and place it on his eyes and forehead.

Sutras 24–25 Under the pretence of preparing some medicine for him he should ask her to do the work for his sake in the following words: "This work must be done by you, and by nobody else." When she wants to go away he should let her go, with an earnest request to come and see him again.

Sutra 26 This device of illness should be continued for three days and three nights.

Sutras 27–28 After this, when she begins coming to see him frequently, he should carry on long conversations with her.

Sutra 29 For, says Ghotakamukha, "though a man loves a girl ever so much, he never succeeds in winning her without a great deal of talking".

Sutra 30 At last, when the man finds the girl completely gained over, he may then begin to enjoy her.

Sutra 31 As for the saying that women grow less timid than usual during the evening and in darkness, and desire congress at those times, do not oppose men then and should only be enjoyed at these hours, it is a matter of talk only.

Sutra 32 When it is impossible for the man to carry on his endeavours alone, he should, by means of the daughter of her nurse, or of a female friend in whom she confides, cause the girl to be brought to him without making known to her his design, and he should then proceed with her in the manner above described.

Sutra 33 Or he should in the beginning send his own female servant to live with the girl as her friend, and should then gain her over by her means.

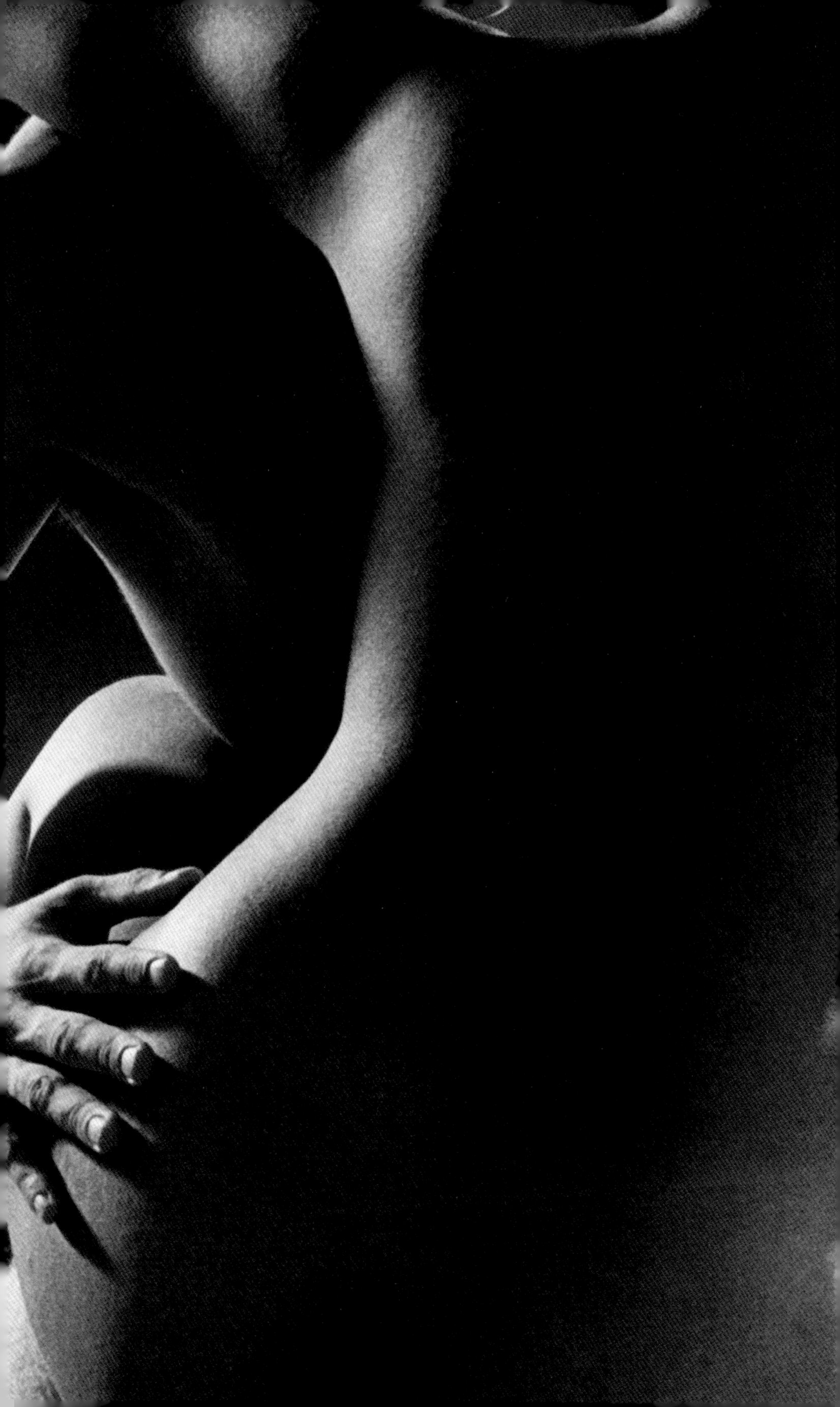

Sutra 34 At last, when he knows the state of her feelings by her outward manner and conduct toward him at religious ceremonies, marriage ceremonies, fairs, festivals, theatres, public assemblies and such occasions, he should begin to enjoy her when she is alone.

Sutra 35 For Vatsyayana lays it down that women, when resorted to at proper times and in proper places, do not turn away from their lovers.

Sutras 36–37 When a girl, possessed of good qualities and well bred, though born in a humble family, or destitute of wealth, and not therefore desired by her equals, or an orphan girl observing the rules of her family and caste, should wish to bring about her own marriage when she comes of age, such a girl should endeavour to win over a strong and good-looking young man, or a person whom she thinks would marry her on account of the weakness of his mind, and even without the consent of his parents.

Sutra 38 She should do this by such means as would endear her to the said person, as well as by frequently seeing and meeting him.

Sutra 39 Her mother also should constantly cause them to meet by means of her female friends, and the daughter of her nurse.

Sutra 40 The girl herself should try to get alone with her beloved in some quiet place, and at odd times should give him flowers, betel nut, betel leaves and perfumes.

Sutras 41–42 She should also show her skill in the practice of the arts, in shampooing, in scratching and in pressing with the nails. She should also talk to him on the subjects he likes best, and discuss with him the ways and means of gaining over and winning the affections of a girl.

Sutras 43–44 But sages say that although the girl loves the man ever so much, she should not offer herself, or make the first overtures, for a girl who does this loses her dignity and is liable to be scorned and rejected.

Sutras 45–46 But when the man shows his wish to enjoy her, she should be favourable to him and should show no change in her demeanour when he embraces her, and should receive all the manifestations of his love as if she were ignorant of the state of his mind.

Sutras 47–49 But when he tries to kiss her she should oppose him; when he begs to be allowed to have sexual intercourse with her she should let him touch her private parts only – and with considerable difficulty; and though importuned by him, she should not yield to him as if of her own accord, but should resist his attempts to have her.

Sutra 50 It is only, moreover, when she is certain that she is truly loved, and that her lover is indeed devoted to her, and will not change his mind, that she should then give herself up to him, and persuade him to marry her quickly.

Sutra 51 After losing her virginity she should tell her confidential friends about it.

Here ends discussion of the efforts of a girl to win over a man.

Sutra 52 There are also some verses on the subject as follows:
"A girl who is much sought after should marry the man that she likes, and whom she thinks would be obedient to her, and capable of giving her pleasure."

Sutra 53 "But when, out of avarice, a girl is married by her parents to a

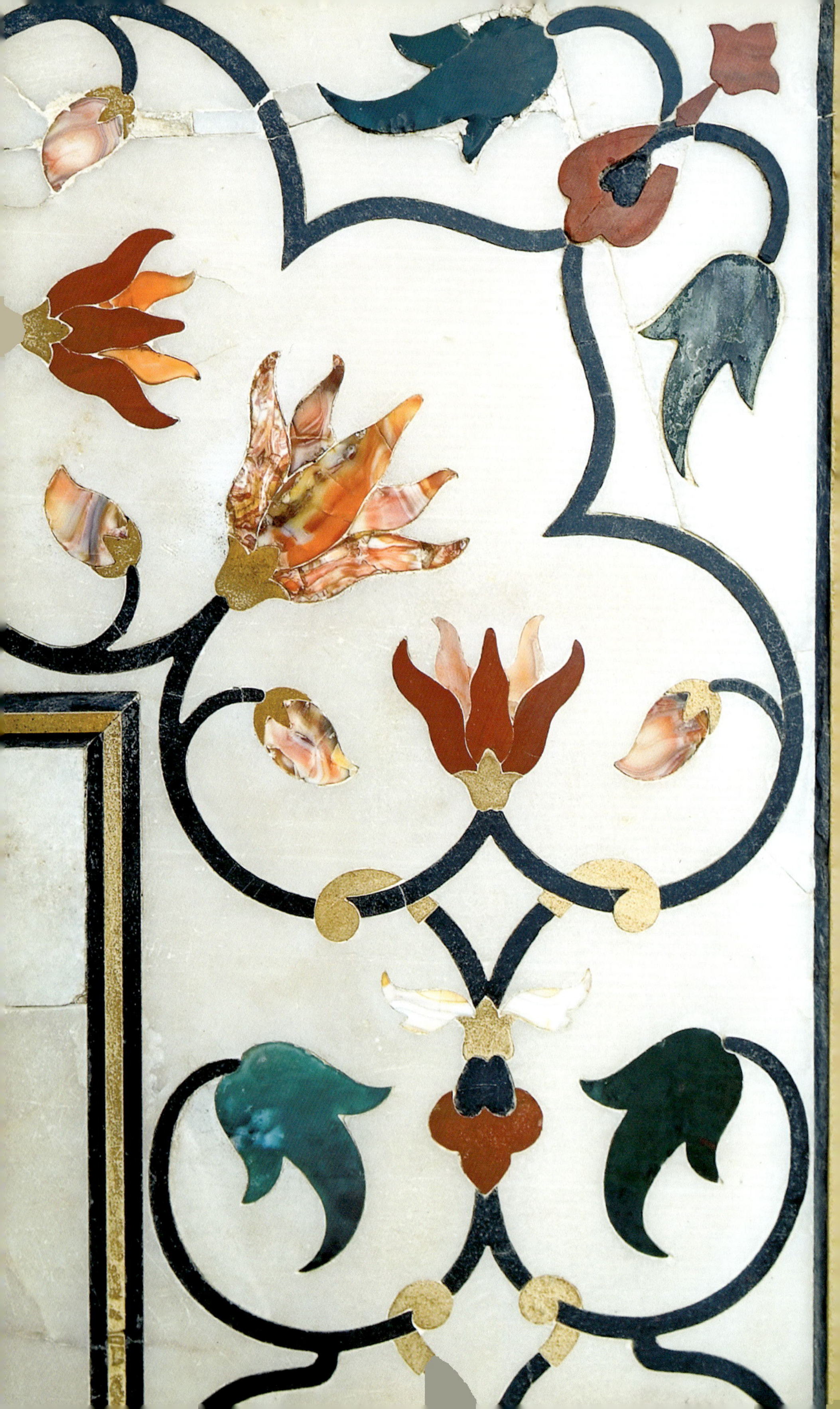

rich man without taking into consideration the character or looks of the bridegroom, or when given to a man who has several wives, she never becomes attached to the man, even though he be endowed with good qualities, obedient to her will, active, strong, healthy and anxious to please her in every way.[5]"

Sutra 54 "A husband who is obedient but yet master of himself, though he be poor and not good looking, is better than one who is common to many women, even though he be handsome and attractive."

Sutra 55 "The wives of rich men, where there are many wives, are not generally attached to their husbands, and are not confidential with them, and even though they possess all the external enjoyments of life, still have recourse to other men."

Sutras 56–58 "A man who is of a low mind, who has fallen from his social position and who is much given to travelling, does not deserve to be married; neither does one who has many wives and children, or one who is devoted to sport and gambling, and who comes to his wife only when he likes."

Sutra 59 "Of all the lovers of a girl he only is her true husband who possesses the qualities that are liked by her, and such a husband only enjoys real superiority over her because he is the husband of love."

Chapter V On certain forms of marriage

Sutra 1 When a girl cannot meet her lover frequently in private, she should send the daughter of her nurse to him, it being understood that she has confidence in her, and had previously gained her over to her interests.

Sutras 2–3 On seeing the man, the daughter of the nurse should, in the course of conversation, describe to him the noble birth, the good disposition, the beauty, talent, skill, knowledge of human nature and affection of the girl in such a way as not to let him suppose that she had been sent by the girl, and should thus create affection for the girl in the heart of the man. To the girl also she should speak of the excellent qualities of the man, especially of those qualities which she knows are pleasing to the girl.

Sutras 4–5 She should, moreover, speak in a disparaging way of the other lovers of the girl, and talk about the avarice and indiscretion of their parents, and the fickleness of their relatives. She should also cite the examples of countless girls from ancient times, such as Sakoontala and others, who, having united themselves with lovers of their own caste and their own choice, attained conjugal happiness ever afterwards in their society.

Sutra 6 And she should also tell of other girls who married into great families, and being troubled by rival wives, became wretched and miserable, and were finally abandoned.

Sutra 7 She should further speak of the good fortune, the continual happiness, the chastity, obedience and affection of the man.

Sutra 8 And if the girl gets amorous about him, she should endeavour to allay her shame[6] and her fear as well as her suspicions about any disaster that might result from her marriage.

Sutra 9 In a word, she should act the whole part of a female messenger by telling the girl all about the man's affection for her, the places he frequented and the endeavours he made to meet her.

Sutra 10 And by frequently repeating, "It will be all right if the man will take you away forcibly and unexpectedly."

The forms of marriage

Sutra 11 When the girl is won over, and acts openly with the man as his wife, he should have fire brought from the house of a Brahmin, and having spread the kusha grass upon the ground, and offered an oblation, he should marry her according to the precepts of the religious law.

Sutras 12–14 After this he should inform his parents of the fact, because it is the opinion of ancient authors that a marriage solemnly contracted in the presence of fire cannot afterwards be set aside.

Sutras 15–16 After the consummation of the marriage, the relations of the man should gradually be made acquainted with the affair, and the relations of the girl should also be informed of it in such a way that they may consent to the marriage, and overlook the manner in which it was brought about, and when this is done they should afterwards be reconciled by affectionate presents and favourable conduct.

Sutra 17 In this manner the man should marry the girl according to the *gandharva* form of marriage.

Sutra 18 When the girl cannot decide, or will not express her readiness to marry, the man should obtain her in any one of the following ways:

Sutra 19 On a fitting occasion, and under some excuse, he should, by means of a female friend with whom he is well acquainted, whom he can trust and who is also well known to the girl's family, get the girl brought unexpectedly to his house, and he should then bring fire from the house of a Brahmin and proceed as described earlier.

Sutra 20 When the marriage of the girl with some other person draws near, the man should disparage the future husband to the utmost in the mind of the mother of the girl.

Sutra 21 Then, having got the girl to come with her mother's consent to a neighbouring house, he should bring fire from the house of a Brahmin and proceed as above.

Sutras 22–23 The man should become a great friend of the brother of the girl – the said brother being of the same age as himself, and addicted to courtesans, and to intrigues with the wives of other people, and he should give him assistance in such matters, and also occasional presents. He should then tell him about his great love for his sister, as young men will sacrifice even their lives for the sake of those who may be of the same age, habits and dispositions as themselves. After this the man should get the girl brought by means of her brother to some secure place, and having brought fire from the house of a Brahmin he should proceed as before.

Sutra 24 The man should, on the occasion of a festival, get the daughter of the nurse to give the girl some intoxicating substance, and then cause her to be brought to some secure place under the pretence of some business; there, having ravished her before she recovers from her intoxication, he should bring fire from the house of a Brahmin and proceed as before.

Sutra 25 The man should, with the connivance of the daughter of the nurse, carry off the girl from her house while she is asleep, and therefore unaware of what is happening, and then, having ravished her before she recovers from her sleep, should bring fire from the house of a Brahmin and proceed as before.

Sutras 26–27 When the girl goes to a garden, or to some village in the neighbourhood, the man should, with his friends, fall on her guards, and having killed them or frightened them away, forcibly carry her off and proceed as before. There are verses on this subject as follows:

Sutra 28 "In all the forms of marriage given in this chapter of this work, the one that precedes is better than the one that follows it on account of its being more in accordance with the commands of religion, and therefore it is only when it is impossible to carry the former into practice that the latter should be resorted to."

Sutra 29 "As the fruit of all good marriages is love, the *gandharva*[7] form of marriage is respected, even though it is formed under unfavourable circumstances, because it fulfils the object sought for. Another cause of the respect accorded to the *gandharva* form of marriage is that it brings forth happiness, causes less trouble in its performance than the other forms of marriage, and is above all the result of previous love."

NOTES

1. The flight of a blue jay on a person's left side is considered a lucky omen when one starts any business; the appearance of a cat before anyone at such a time is looked on as a bad omen. There are many omens of this kind.
2. Such as the throbbing of the right eye of men and the left eye of women.
3. Before anything is begun it is a custom to go early in the morning to a neighbour's house and overhear the first words that may be spoken in his family, and according to whether the words heard are of good or bad import, to draw an inference as to the success or failure of the undertaking.
4. A disease consisting of any glandular enlargement in any part of the body.
5. There is a good deal of truth in the last few observations. Woman is a monogamous animal and loves but one, and likes to feel herself alone in the affections of one man, and cannot bear rivals. It may also be taken as a general rule that women either married to, or kept by, rich men love them for their wealth but not for themselves.
6. About this, see a story on the fatal effects of love in *Early Ideas; a Group of Hindoo Stories*, collected and collated by Anaryan (W.H. Allen and Co., London, 1881, page 114).
7. About the *gandharvavivaha* form of marriage, see the note to page 28 of R.F. Burton's *Vickram and the Vampire; or Tales of Hindu Devilry* (Longmans, Green and Co., London, 1870). This form of matrimony was recognized by the ancient Hindus and is frequent in books. It is a kind of Scottish wedding – ultra-Caledonian – taking place by mutual consent without any form or ceremony. The *gandharvas* are heavenly minstrels of Indra's court, who are supposed to be mistresses.

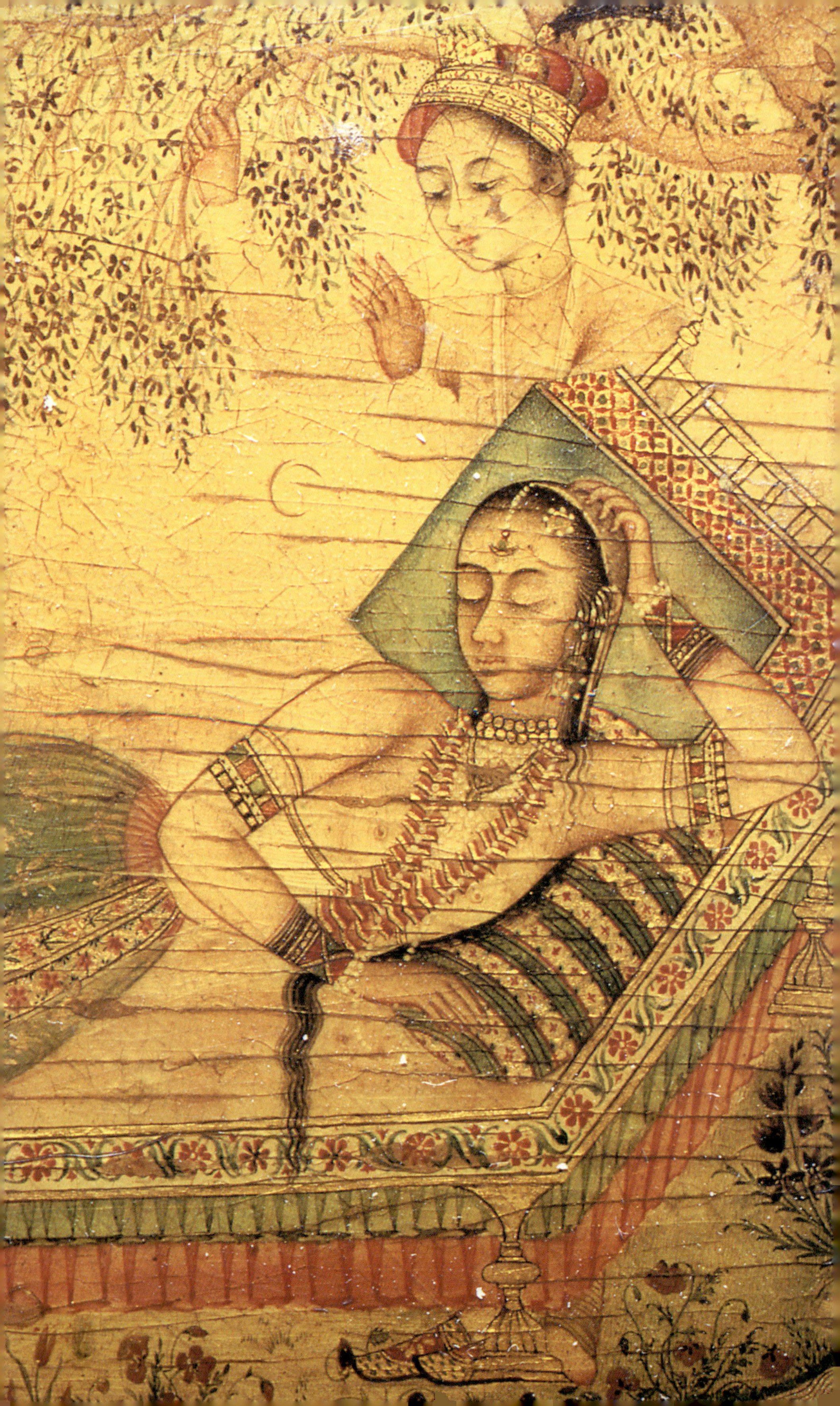

Part Four: On the Duties and Privileges of a Wife

Chapter I The manner of living of a virtuous woman, and her behaviour during her husband's absence

Sutra 1 A virtuous woman, who has affection for her husband, should act in conformity with his wishes as if he were a divine being,

Sutra 2 And with his consent she should take upon herself the whole care of his family.

Sutra 3 She should keep their house well cleaned, arrange flowers of various kinds in different parts of it, and make the floor smooth and polished so as to give the whole a neat and becoming appearance. She should surround the house with a garden, and place ready in it all the materials required for the morning, noon and evening sacrifices. Moreover she should herself revere the sanctuary of the household gods.

Sutra 4 As Gonardiya says, "nothing so much attracts the heart of a householder to his wife as a careful observance of the things mentioned above".

Sutra 5 Toward the parents, relations, friends, sisters and servants of her husband she should behave in a fitting way.

Sutras 6–7 In the garden she should plant beds of green vegetables, bunches of sugar cane, clumps of the fig tree, garcinia, the mustard plant, the parsley plant and the fennel plant. Clusters of various flowers such as the water chestnut [*Trapa bispinosa*], jasmine, wild jasmine, crepe jasmine, yellow amaranth, the china rose [hibiscus] and others, should likewise be planted, together with the fragrant grass *Andropogon schoenanthus*, and the fragrant root of the plant *Andropogon miricatus*.

Sutra 8 She should also have seats and arbours made in the garden, in the middle of which a well, tank, or pool should be dug.

Sutra 9 The wife should avoid the company of roguish women, female beggars, Buddhist mendicants and fortune-tellers, and witches.

Sutra 10 Foodwise she should always consider what her husband likes and dislikes, which things are good for him and which are injurious.

Sutra 11 When she hears the sounds of his footsteps coming home she should at once get up and be ready to do whatever he may command her.

Sutra 12 She should either order her female servant to wash his feet or wash them herself.

Sutra 13 When going anywhere with her husband, she should put on her ornaments.

Sutra 14 She should not either give or accept invitations without her husband's consent.

Sutra 15 She should obtain his consent to attend marriages and sacrifices, or sit in the company of female friends, or visit temples.

Sutra 16 And if she wants to engage in any kind of games or sports, she should not do it against his will.

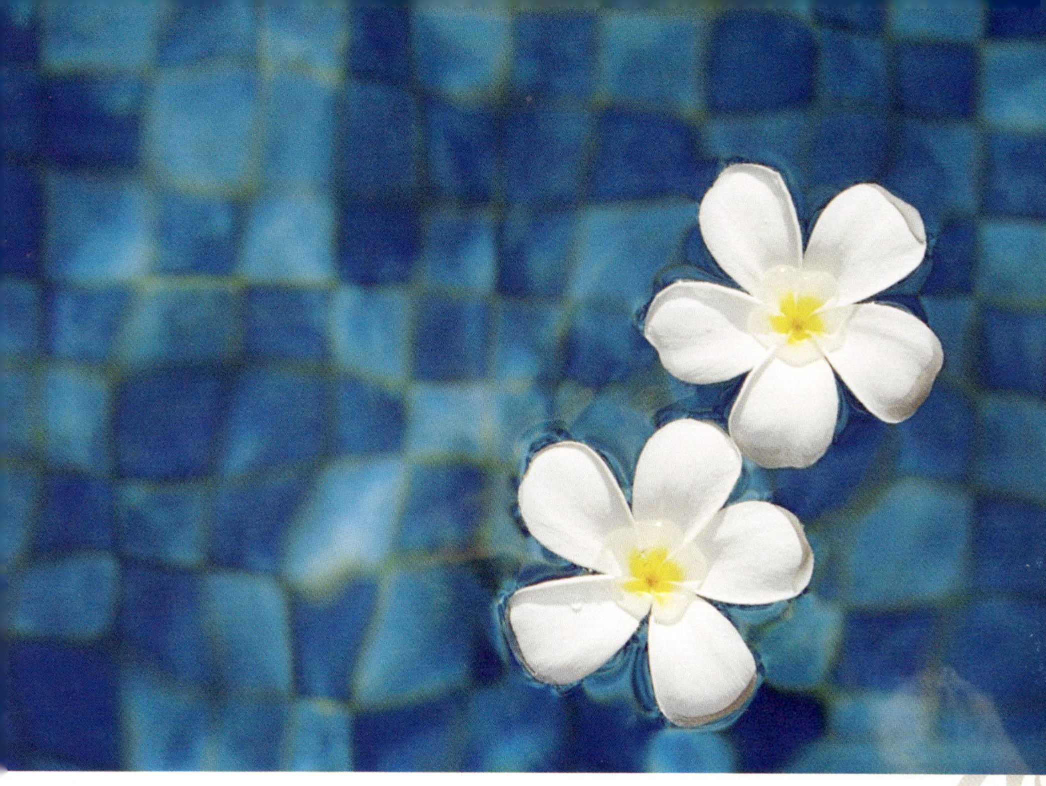

Sutra 17 In the same way she should always sit down after him, and get up before him, and should never wake him when he is asleep.

Sutra 18 The kitchen should be situated in a quiet place well within the house, so as not to be accessible to strangers, and should always look clean.

Sutra 19 In the event of any misconduct on the part of her husband, she should not blame him excessively, though she be a little displeased.

Sutra 20 She should not use abusive language toward him, but rebuke him with conciliatory words, whether he be in the company of friends or alone.

Sutra 21 Moreover, she should not be a scold, for, says Gonardiya, "there is no cause of dislike on the part of a husband so great as this characteristic in a wife".

Sutra 22 She should avoid bad expressions, sulky looks, talking while facing away, standing in the doorway, looking at passers-by, conversing in the pleasure groves, and remaining in a secluded place for a long time.

Sutra 23 And finally she should always keep her body, her teeth, her hair, and everything belonging to her, tidy, sweet and clean.

Sutra 24 When the wife wants to attract her husband she should dress with many ornaments, various kinds of flowers, a cloth decorated with different colours, and some sweet-smelling ointments or unguents.

Sutra 25 But her everyday dress should be composed of a thin, close-textured cloth, a few ornaments and flowers, and a little scent, not too much.

Sutra 26 She should also observe the fasts and vows of her husband, and when he tries to prevent her doing this, she should persuade him to let her do it.

Sutra 27 At appropriate times of the year, and when they happen to be cheap, she should buy clay, bamboo, firewood, leather and iron pots, as well as salt and oil.

Sutra 28 Fragrant substances, vessels made of the fruit of the plant Sweet Indrajao [*Wrightia antidysenterica*], or oval-leaved *wrightia*, medicines, and other things which are always wanted, should be obtained when required and kept in a secret place in the house.

Sutra 29 She should buy and sow during the proper seasons the seeds of the radish, potato, common beet, Indian wormwood, mango,

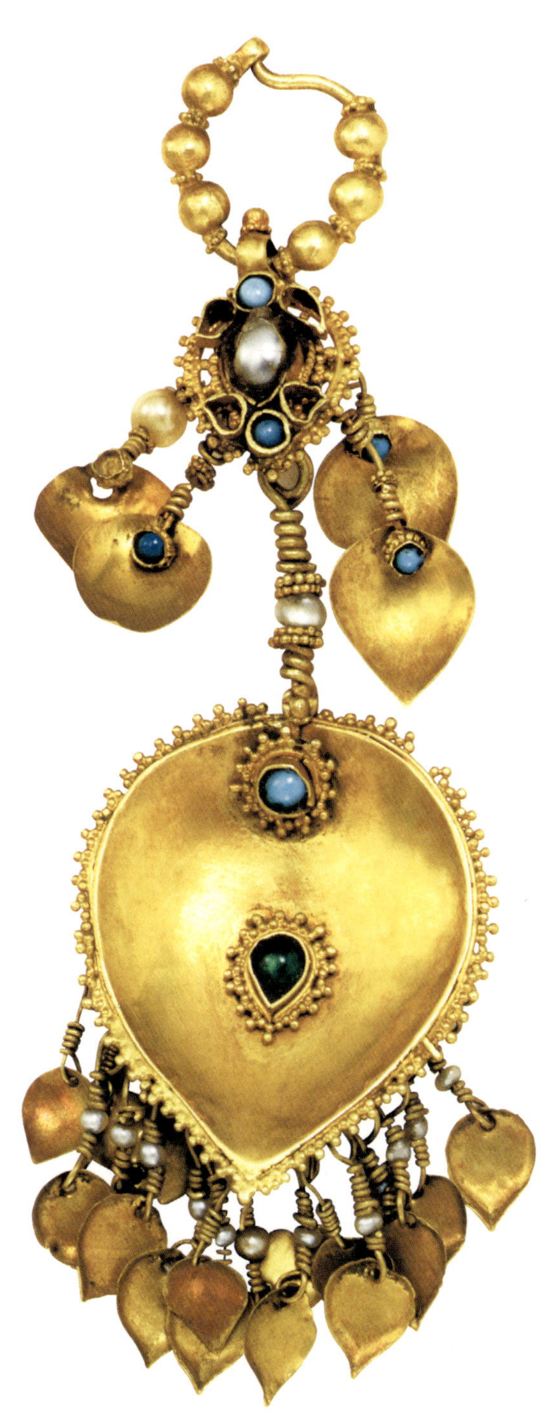

cucumber, eggplant, *kushmanda*, pumpkin gourd, *surana*, *Bignonia indica*, sandalwood, *Premna spinosa*, garlic, onion and other vegetables.

Sutra 30 The wife should not divulge to strangers the amount of her wealth, nor the secrets which her husband has confided to her.

Sutra 31 She should surpass all the women of her own rank in life in her cleverness, her appearance, her knowledge of cookery, her pride and her manner of serving her husband.

Sutra 32 Annual income should be budgeted and expenditure controlled.

Sutra 33 The milk that remains after meals should be turned into ghee or clarified butter. Oil and sugar should be prepared at home; spinning and weaving should also be done there; and a store of ropes and cords, and barks of trees for twisting into ropes, should be kept. She should also attend to the pounding and cleaning of rice, using its grain and chaff in some way or other. She should pay the salaries of the servants, look after the tilling of the fields, and the keeping of the flocks and herds, superintend the making of vehicles, and take care of the rams, cocks, quails, parrots, starlings, cuckoos, peacocks, monkeys and deer; and finally adjust the income and expenditure of the day.

Sutra 34 Worn-out clothes should be given to those servants who have done good work, in order to show them that their services have been appreciated, or they may be put to some other use.

Sutra 35 The vessels in which wine is prepared, as well as those in which it is kept, should be carefully looked after, and put away at the proper time. All sales and purchases should also be well attended to.

Sutra 36 She should welcome her husband's friends by presenting them with flowers, ointment, incense, betel leaves and betel nut.

Sutra 37 Her parents-in-law she should treat as they deserve, always remaining dependent on their will, never contradicting them, speaking to them moderately, and never laughing loudly in their presence.

Sutra 38 She should behave with their friends and enemies as she would with her own.

Sutra 39 In addition to the above she should not be vain, or too much taken up with her enjoyments.

Sutra 40 She should be liberal toward her servants, and reward them at holidays and festival time.

Sutra 41 She should not give away anything without first making it known to her husband.

Sutra 42 Thus ends the manner of living of a virtuous woman.

Sutra 43 During her husband's absence on a journey the virtuous woman should wear only her auspicious ornaments, and observe religious fasts. While anxious to hear the news of her husband, she should still look after her household affairs.

Sutras 44–45 At night she should sleep near the elder women of the house, and act in accordance with their wishes.

Sutras 46–48 She should safeguard the things that are liked by her husband, and continue any works that have been begun by him.

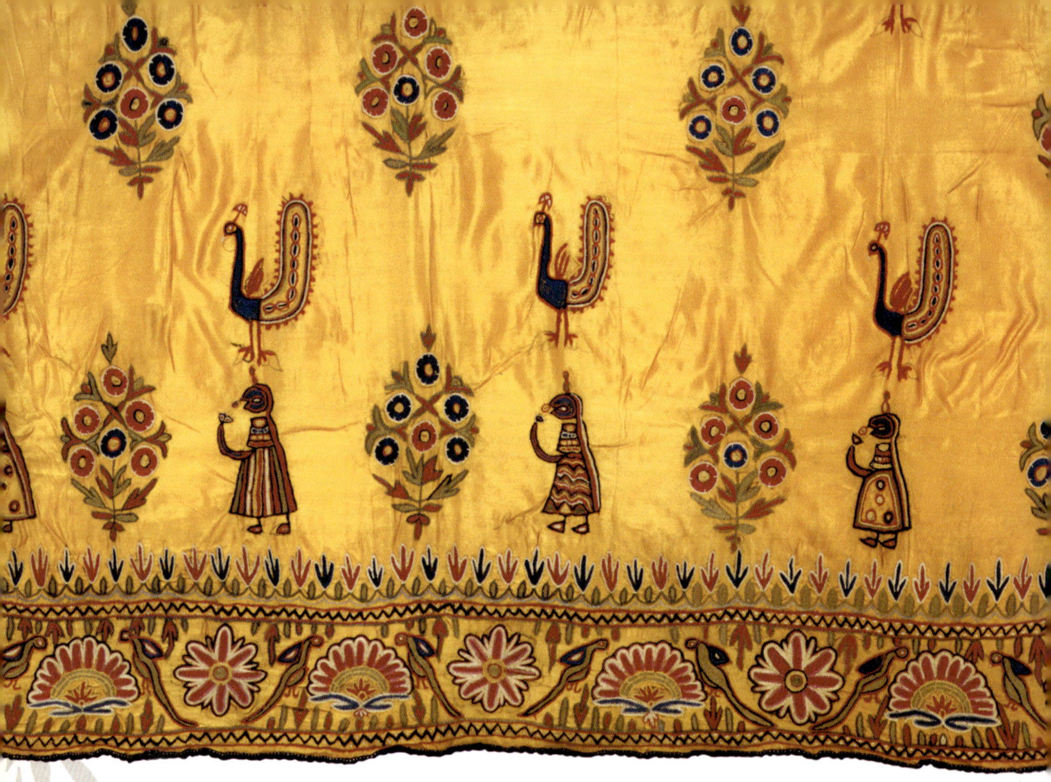

Sutra 49 To the abode of her relations she should not go except when there is a festival or a death.

Sutra 50 And upon such an occasion she should go in her usual travelling dress, accompanied by her husband's servants, and not remain there for a long time.

Sutra 51 The fasts and feasts should be observed with the consent of the elders of the house.

Sutra 52 The household resources should be increased by making purchases and sales economically, and by using honest servants, superintended by herself.

The household income should be increased, and the expenditure diminished, as much as possible.

Sutra 53 And when her husband returns from his journey, she should receive him at first in her ordinary clothes, so that he may know in what way she has lived during his absence, and she should bring to him some presents, as well as materials for worship.

Thus ends the part relating to the behaviour of a wife during the absence of her husband on a journey.

Sutra 54 There are also some verses on the subject as follows:

Sutra 55 "The wife, whether she be a woman of noble family, or a virgin widow[1] remarried, or a concubine, should lead a chaste life, devoted to her husband, and doing everything for his welfare."

Sutra 56 Women acting thus acquire Dharma, Artha and Kama, obtain a high position, and generally keep their husbands devoted to them.

Chapter II On the conduct of the elder wife toward the other wives of her husband, and on that of a younger wife toward the elder ones; also on the conduct of a virgin widow remarried; of a wife disliked by her husband; of the women in the king's harem; and lastly on the conduct of a husband toward many wives

Sutra 1 The reasons for remarrying during the lifetime of the wife are as follows:

The folly or ill-temper of the wife
Her husband's dislike of her
The desire to have offspring
The successive birth of daughters
The sensuous weakness of the husband

Sutra 2 From the very beginning, a wife should endeavour to attract the heart of her husband, by continually showing to him her devotion, her good temper and her wisdom.

Sutra 3 If however she bears him no children, she should herself tell her husband to marry another woman.

Sutras 4–5 And when the second wife is married, and brought to the house, the first wife should give her a position superior to her own, and look upon her as a sister.

Sutra 6 In the morning the elder wife should forcibly make the younger one decorate herself in the presence of their husband, and should not mind all the husband's favour being given to her.

Sutras 7–10 If the younger wife does anything to displease her husband the elder one should not neglect her, but should always be ready to give her most careful advice, and should teach her to do various things in the presence of her husband.

Sutras 11–15 Her children she should treat as her own, her attendants she should look upon with even more regard than her own servants, her friends she should cherish with love and kindness, and her relations with great honour.

Sutra 16 When there are many co-wives, the elder wife should associate with the one who is immediately next to her in rank and age.

Sutras 17–18 When the elder wife finds that the husband favours the new wife too much she should instigate a quarrel betwen the wife who has recently been her husband's favourite and the one who is the present favourite.

Sutra 19 After this she should sympathize with the former, and having collected all the other wives together, she should get them to denounce the favourite as a scheming and wicked woman, without herself quarrelling in any way.

Sutras 20–21 If the favourite wife happens to quarrel with the husband, then the elder wife should take her part and give her false encouragement, and thus cause the quarrel to be increased.

Sutra 22 If there be only a small quarrel between the two, the elder wife should do all she can to work it up into a large quarrel.

Sutra 23 But if after all this she finds the husband still continues to love his favourite wife she should then change her tactics, and endeavour to bring about a conciliation between them, so as to avoid her husband's displeasure.

Thus ends the conduct of the elder wife.

Sutra 24 The younger wife should regard the elder wife of her husband as her mother.

Sutras 25–26 She should not give gifts, even to her own relations, without her knowledge.

Sutra 27 She should tell her everything about herself, and not approach her husband without her permission.

Sutra 28 Whatever is told to her by the elder wife she should not reveal.

Sutra 29–30 She should take care of the children of the senior even more than of her own.

Sutra 31 When alone with her husband she should serve him well, but should not tell him of the pain she suffers from the existence of a rival.

Sutras 32–33 She may also obtain secretly from her husband some marks of his particular regard for her, and may tell him that she lives only for him, and for the regard that he has for her.

Sutra 34 She should never reveal her love for her husband, nor her husband's love for her, to any person, either in pride or in anger.

Sutra 35 A wife that divulges secrets displeases her husband.

Sutra 36 Gonardiya says that a younger wife seeking to obtain the regard of her husband should always do so in private, for fear of the elder wife.

Sutra 37 If the elder wife be disliked by her husband, or be childless, the younger wife should sympathize with her, and should ask her husband to do the same.

Sutra 38 But the younger wife should surpass the elder in leading the life of a chaste woman.

Thus ends the conduct of the younger wife toward the elder.

Sutra 39 A widow in poor circumstances, or of a weak nature, and who again allies herself to a man, is called a widow remarried.

Sutras 40–41 The followers of Babhravya say that a virgin widow should not marry a person whom she may have to leave on account of his bad character, or of his being devoid of gentlemanly qualities, obliging her to seek another husband.

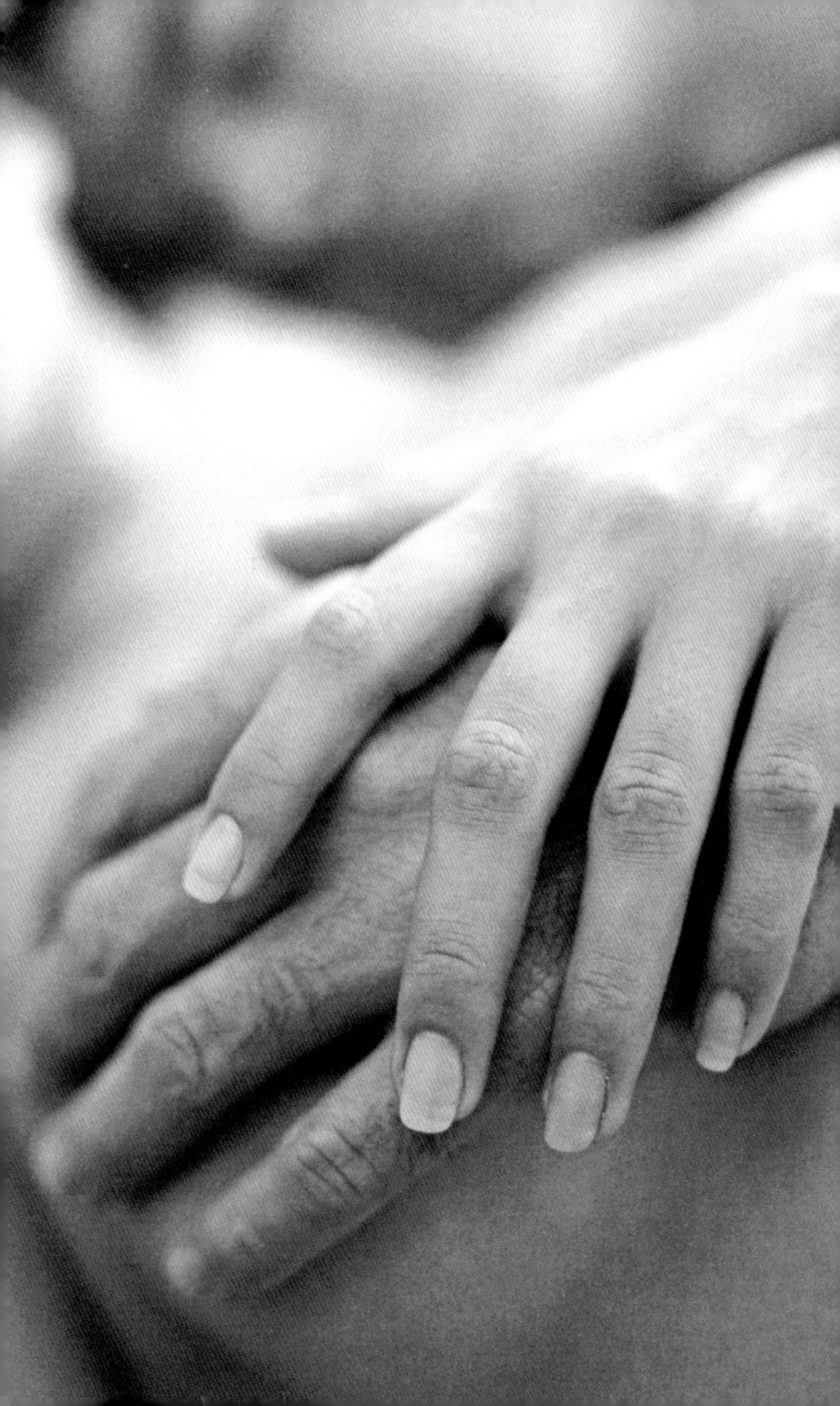

Sutra 42 Gonardiya is of the opinion that because a widow remarries to seek happiness, and as happiness is secured by the husband having excellent qualities, joined to love of enjoyment, it is better to secure a person endowed with such qualities in the first instance.

Sutra 43 Vatsyayana, however, thinks that a widow may marry any person that she likes, and that she thinks will suit her.

Sutra 44 At the time of her marriage the widow should obtain from her husband the money to pay the cost of drinking parties and picnics with her relations, and to give them and her friends kindly gifts and presents; or she may do these things at her own cost if she likes.

Sutra 45 In the same way, she may wear either her husband's ornaments or her own.

Sutra 46 As to the presents of affection mutually exchanged between the husband and herself, there is no fixed rule about them.

Sutra 47 If after marriage she leaves her husband of her own accord, she should restore to him whatever he may have given her, with the exception of the mutual presents. If, however, she is driven out of the house by her husband she should not return anything to him.

Sutras 48–52 After her marriage she should live in the house of her husband like one of the chief members of the family, but she should treat the other ladies of the family with kindness, the servants with generosity, and all the friends of the house cordially.

Sutra 53 She should show that she is better acquainted with the sixty-four arts than the other ladies of the house, and in any quarrels with her husband she should not rebuke him severely, but in private do everything that he wishes and make use of her knowledge of the sixty-four ways of enjoyment.

Sutras 54–55 She should be obliging to the other wives of her husband, and to their children she should give presents.

Sutra 56 Behave as their mistress, and make ornaments and playthings for their use.

Sutras 57–58 She should confide more in the friends and servants of her husband than in his other wives.

Sutra 59 Finally, she should like drinking parties, going to picnics, attending fairs and festivals, and carrying out all kinds of games and amusements.

Thus ends the conduct of a virgin widow remarried.

Sutra 60 A woman who is disliked by her husband, and annoyed and distressed by his other wives, should associate with the wife who is liked most by her husband, and who serves him more than the others.

Sutras 61–62 And she should teach her all the arts with which she is acquainted.

Sutras 63–64 She should act as the nurse to her husband's children, and having won over his friends to her side, through them she should convey her devotion to him.

Sutras 65–66 In religious ceremonies she should be a leader, likewise in vows and fasts, and she should not hold too good an opinion of herself.

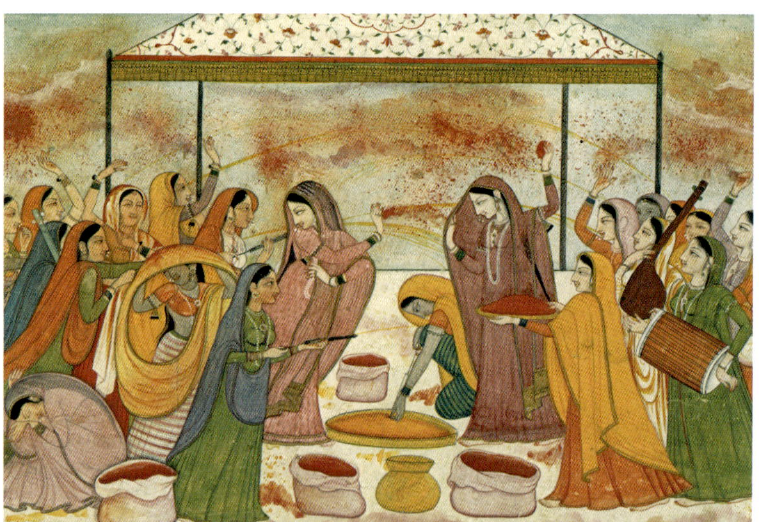

Sutra 67 When her husband is lying on his bed she should only go near him when it is agreeable to him.

Sutra 68 She should never rebuke him, or show obstinacy in any way.

Sutra 69 If her husband happens to quarrel with any of his other wives, she should reconcile them to each other.

Sutra 70 If he desires to see any woman secretly, she should manage to bring about the meeting between them.

Sutra 71 She should make herself acquainted with the weak points of her husband's character, but always keep them secret, and on the whole behave herself in such a way as may lead him to look upon her as a good and devoted wife.

Here ends the conduct of a wife disliked by her husband.

Sutra 72 The above sections will show how all the women of the king's harem are to behave, and therefore we shall now speak separately about the king.

Sutra 73 The female attendants in the harem (called severally *kanchukiyas*,[2] *mahallarikas*,[3] and *mahallikas*[4]) should bring flowers, ointments and clothes from the king's wives to the king.

Sutra 74 Having received these things, the king should give them as presents to the servants, along with the things worn by him the previous day.

Sutra 75 In the afternoon the king, having dressed and put on his ornaments, should interview the women of the harem, who should also be dressed and decorated with jewels.

Sutra 76 Then, having given to each of them such a place and such respect as may suit the occasion, and as they may deserve, he should carry on a cheerful conversation with them.

Sutra 77 After that he should see those of his wives who are virgin widows remarried,

Sutras 78–79 And after them the concubines and dancing girls. All of these should be visited in their own private rooms.

Sutras 80–81 When the king rises from his noonday sleep, the woman whose duty it is to inform the king about the wife who is to spend the night with him should come to him accompanied by the female attendants of anyone who may have been accidentally passed over as her turn arrived, and of anyone who may have been unwell at the time of her turn. These attendants should place before the king the ointments and unguents sent by each of these wives, marked with the seal of her ring, and their names and their reasons for sending the ointments should be told to the king. After this the king accepts the ointment of one of them, who is then informed that it has been accepted and that her day has been settled.[5]

Sutra 82 At festivals, singing parties and exhibitions, all the wives of the king should be treated with respect and served with drinks.

Sutra 83 But the women of the harem should not be allowed to go out alone, neither should any women outside the harem be allowed to enter it except those whose character is well known. And, lastly, the work which the king's wives have to do should not be too fatiguing.

Sutra 84 Thus ends the conduct of the king toward the women of the harem, and of their own conduct.

Sutra 85 A man marrying many wives should act fairly toward them all. He should neither disregard nor pass over their faults,

Sutras 86–87 And he should not reveal to one wife the love, passion, bodily blemishes and confidential reproaches of the other. No opportunity should be given to any one of them to speak to him about their rivals, and if one of them should begin to speak ill of another, he should chide her and tell her that she has exactly the same blemishes in her character.

Sutras 88–89 One of them he should please by secret confidence, another by secret respect, and another by secret flattery; and he should please them all by going to gardens, by amusements, by presents, by honouring their relations, by telling them secrets and by loving unions.

Sutra 90 A young woman who is of a good temper, and who conducts herself according to the holiest precepts, wins her husband's devotion and obtains a superiority over her rivals.

Thus ends the conduct of a husband toward many wives.

NOTES

1. This probably refers to a girl married in her infancy, or when very young, and whose husband had died before she arrived at the age of puberty.
2. A name given to the maidservants of kings in ancient times, on account of their always keeping their breasts covered with a cloth called a *kanchuki*. It was customary in those days for the maidservants to cover their breasts with a cloth while the queens kept their breasts uncovered. This custom can be seen in the paintings in the Ajanta caves.
3. Meaning a superior woman; thus it would seem that a *mahallarika* must be a person in authority over the maidservants of the house.
4. This also appertained to the rank of women employed in the harem. In later times this place was given to eunuchs.
5. As kings generally had many wives it was usual for them to enjoy their wives by turns. But as it happened sometimes that some of them lost their turns owing to the king's absence, or their being unwell, then in such cases the women whose turns had been passed over, and those whose turns had come, used to have a sort of lottery, and the ointments of all the claimants were sent to the king, who accepted the ointment of one of them, and thus settled the question.

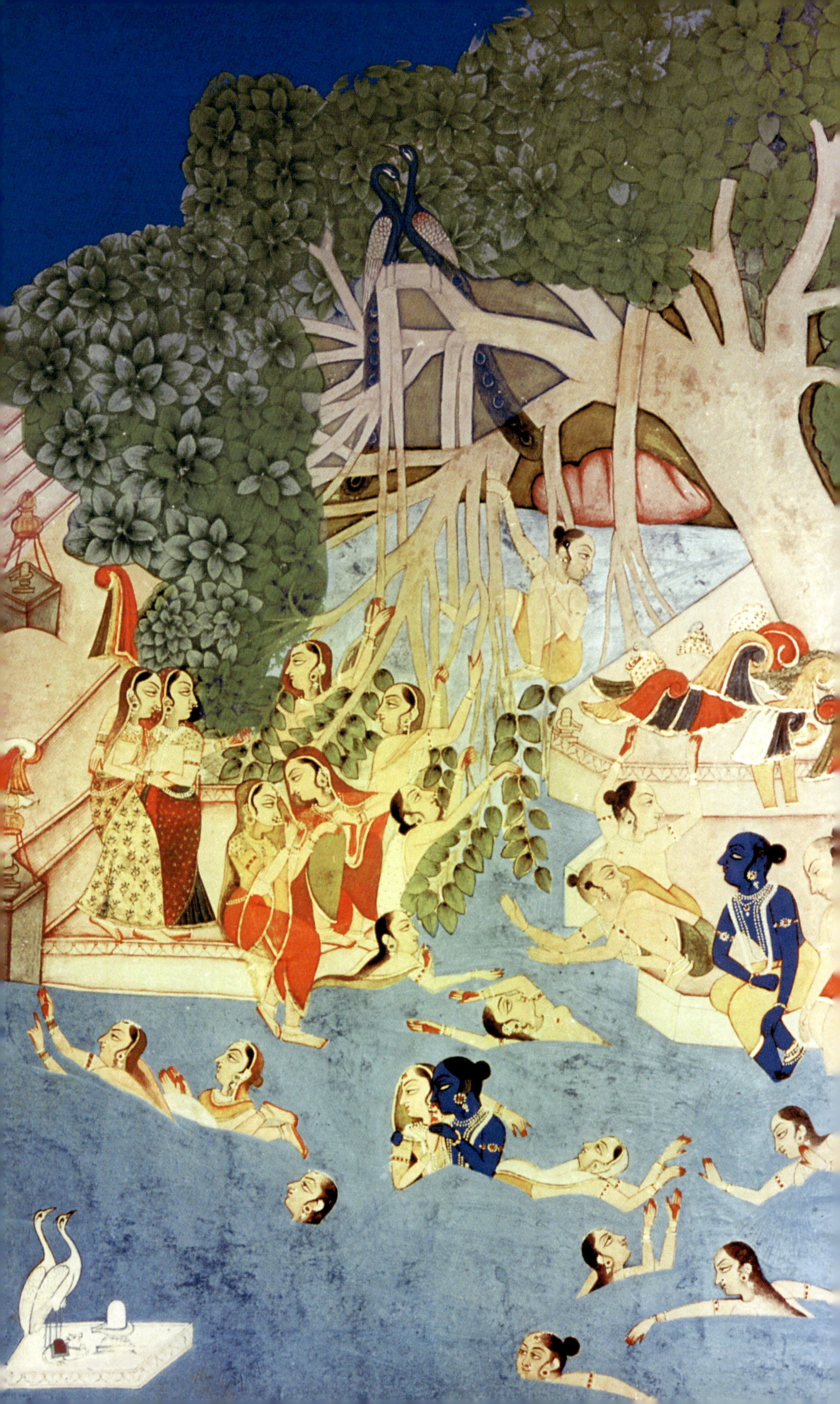

Part Five: On Relations with Wives of Other Men

Chapter I The characteristics of men and women; the reasons why women reject the addresses of men; about men who have success with women; and about women who are easily won over

Sutra 1–2 The wives of other people may be resorted to on the occasions already described in this work [see pages 37–43], but the possibility of their acquisition, their fitness for cohabitation, the danger to oneself in uniting with them, and the future effect of these unions, should all be examined first.

Sutra 3 A man may resort to the wife of another for the purpose of saving his own life, when he perceives that his love for her proceeds from one degree of intensity to another.

Sutras 4–5 These degrees are ten in number, and are distinguished by the following marks:

Love of the eye
Attachment of the mind
Constant reflection
Destruction of sleep
Emaciation of the body
Turning away from objects of enjoyment
Removal of shame
Madness
Fainting
Death

Sutra 6 Ancient authors say that a man should recognize the disposition, truthfulness, purity and will of a young woman – and also the intensity, or weakness, of her passions – from the form of her body, and from her characteristic marks and signs.

Sutra 7 But Vatsyayana is of opinion that the forms of bodies, and the characteristic marks or signs, are not enough to go by, and that women should be judged by their conduct, the outward expression of their thoughts, and the movements of their bodies.

Sutra 8 As a general rule Gonikaputra says that a woman falls in love with every handsome man she sees, and so does every man at the sight of a beautiful woman, but frequently they do not take any further steps, owing to various considerations.

Sutra 9 In love the following circumstances are peculiar to the woman.

Sutra 10 She loves without regard to right or wrong, and does not try to win over a man simply for the attainment of some particular purpose.

Sutras 11–12 Moreover, when a man first approaches her she naturally shrinks from him, even though she may not be averse to union with him. But when the attempts to woo her are repeated and renewed, she at last consents.

Sutra 13 On the other hand, a man who is attracted to a beautiful woman conquers his feelings for union due to moral considerations.

Sutra 14 And although his thoughts are often on the woman, he does not yield, despite attempts she may make to win him over.

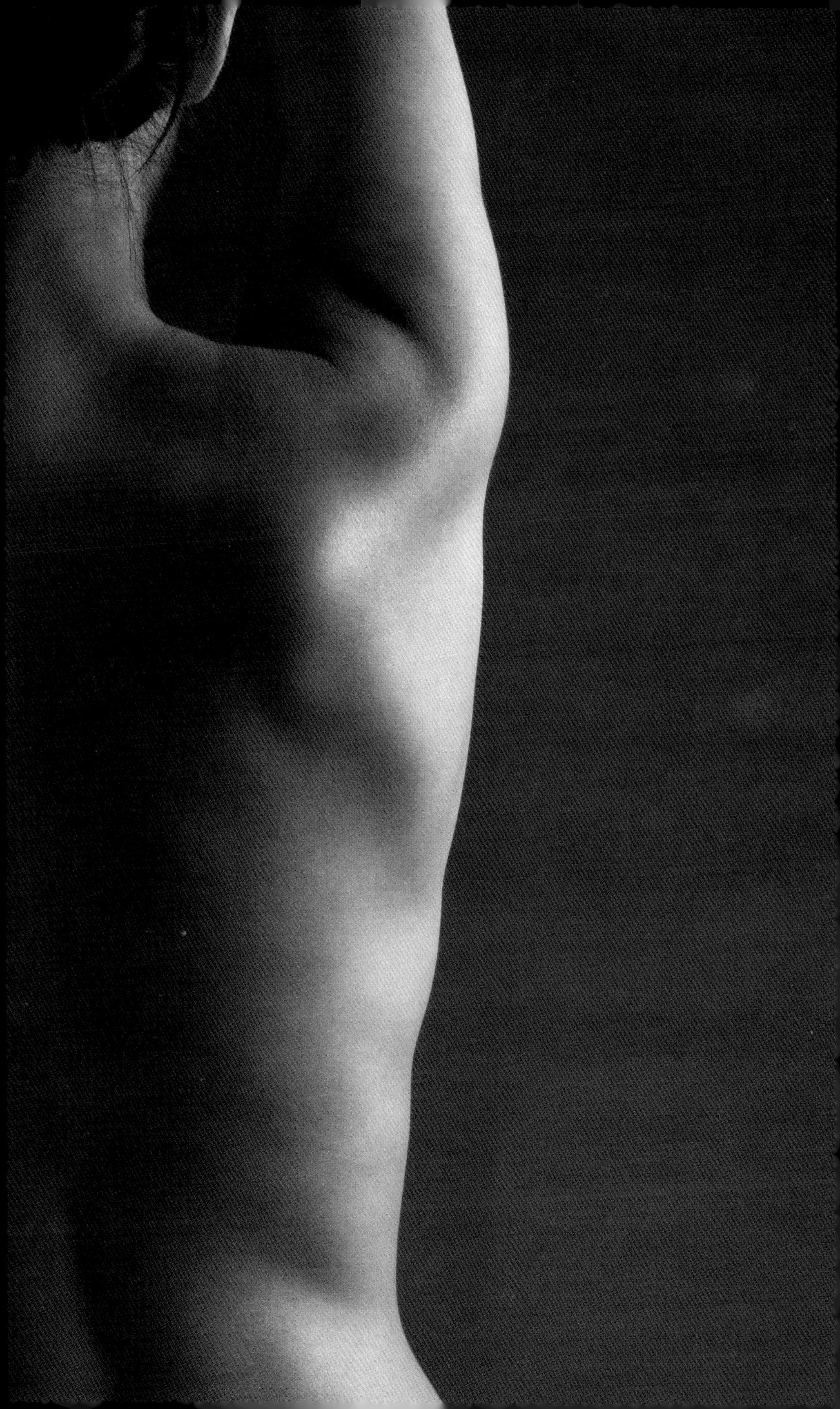

Sutra 15 He sometimes makes an attempt or effort to win the object of his affections, and, having failed, he leaves her alone for the future.

Sutra 16 In the same way, when a woman has been won over he often becomes indifferent. It is said that a man does not care for what is easily gained, and desires a thing which can only be obtained with difficulty.

Sutra 17 The causes of a woman rebuffing a man are as follows:

Sutra 18 Affection for her husband.

Sutra 19 Desire for lawful progeny.

Sutra 20 Want of opportunity.

Sutra 21 Anger at being addressed by the man in too familiar a way.

Sutra 22 Difference in age.

Sutra 23 Want of certainty about the man's sentiments.

Sutra 24 Thinking that the man may be attached to some other person.

Sutra 25 Fear of the man's not keeping his intentions secret.

Sutra 26 Thinking that the man is too devoted to his friends, and has too great a regard for them.

Sutra 27 The apprehension that he is not in earnest.

Sutra 28 Bashfulness on account of his being an illustrious man.

Sutra 29 Fear on account of his being powerful, or possessed of too impetuous passion, in the case of the deer woman.

Sutra 30 Bashfulness on account of his being too clever.

Sutra 31 The thought of having once lived with him on friendly terms only.

Sutra 32 Contempt of his want of knowledge of the world.

Sutra 33 Distrust of his low character.

Sutra 34 Disgust at his want of perception of her love for him.

Sutra 35 In the case of an elephant woman, the thought that he is a hare man, or a man of weak passion.

Sutra 36 Compassion lest anything should befall him on account of his passion.

Sutra 37 Despair at her own imperfections.

Sutra 38 Fear of discovery.

Sutra 39 Disillusion at seeing his grey hair or shabby appearance.

Sutra 40 Her suspicion that he may be employed by her husband to test her chastity.

Sutra 41–42 The thought that he has too much regard for moral considerations.

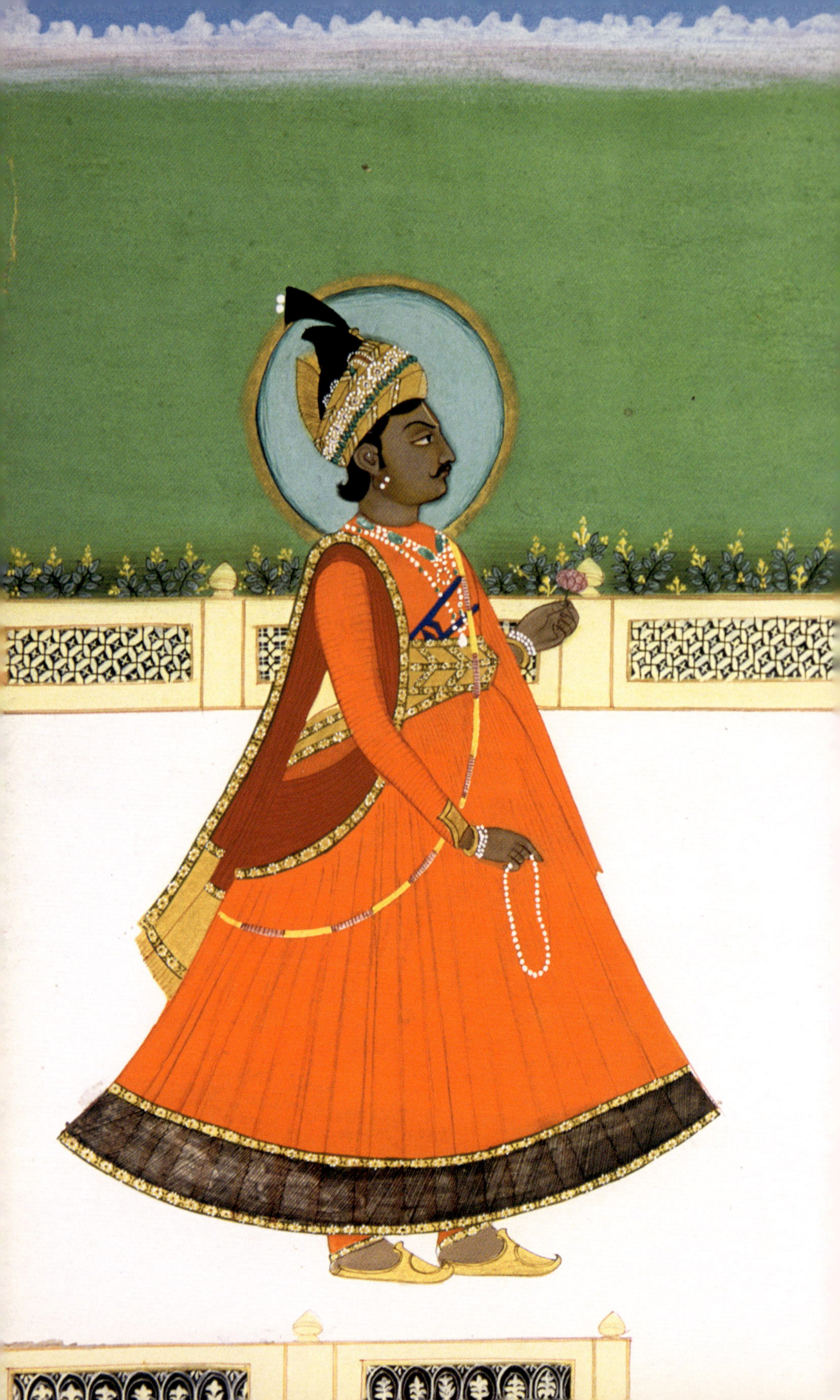

Sutra 43 Whichever of the above causes a man may detect, he should endeavour to remove it from the very beginning.

Sutra 44 Thus, the bashfulness that may arise from his greatness or ability, he should remove by showing his love and affection for her.

Sutra 45 The difficulty of the want of opportunity, or of his inaccessibility, he should remove by showing her some remedies.

Sutra 46 The excessive respect entertained by the woman for him should be removed by making himself very familiar.

Sutra 47 The difficulties that arise from his being thought a low character he should remove by showing his valour and his wisdom.

Sutras 48–49 Those that come from neglect, by giving her extra attention; and those that arise from fear, by giving her proper encouragement.

Sutras 50–51 The following are the men who generally obtain success with women:

Men well versed in the science of love
Men skilled in telling stories
Men acquainted with women from their childhood
Men who have secured their confidence
Men who send presents to them
Men who talk well
Men who do things that they like
Men who have not loved other women previously
Men who act as messengers
Men who know their weak points

Men who are desired by good women
Men who are united with their female friends
Men who are good looking
Men who have been brought up with them
Men who are their neighbours
Men who are devoted to sexual pleasures, even though these be with their own servants
The lovers of the daughters of their nurse
Men who have recently been married
Men who like picnics and pleasure parties
Men who are liberal
Men who are celebrated for being very strong (bull men)
Enterprising and brave men
Men who surpass their husbands in learning and good looks, in good qualities, and in liberality
Men who dress and behave in an aristocratic manner

Sutra 52 The following are the women who are easily won over:
Women who stand at the doors of their houses
Women who are always looking out on the street
Women who sit conversing in their neighbour's house
A woman who is always staring at you
A female messenger
A woman who looks sideways at you
A woman whose husband has taken another wife without just cause
A woman who hates her husband, or who is hated by him
A woman who has nobody to look after her, or keep her in check
A woman who has not had any children
A woman whose family or caste is not well known
A woman whose children are dead
A woman who is very fond of society

A woman who is apparently very affectionate with her husband
The wife of an actor
A widow
A poor woman
A woman fond of enjoyments
The wife of a man with many younger brothers
A vain woman
A woman whose husband is inferior to her in rank or abilities
A woman who is proud of her skill in the arts
A woman disturbed in mind by the folly of her husband
A woman who has been married in her infancy to a rich man, and not liking him when she grows up, desires a man possessing a disposition, talents and wisdom suitable to her own tastes
A woman who is slighted by her husband without any cause
A woman who is not respected by other women of the same rank or beauty as herself
A woman whose husband is devoted to travelling
The wife of a jeweler
A jealous woman
A covetous woman
An immoral woman
A barren woman
A lazy woman
A cowardly woman
A humpbacked woman
A dwarfish woman
A deformed woman
A vulgar woman
An ill-smelling woman
A sick woman
An old woman

Sutra 53 There are also two verses on the subject as follows:

"Desire, which springs from nature, and which is increased by art, and from which all danger is taken away by wisdom, becomes firm and secure."

Sutra 54 "A clever man, depending on his own ability, and observing carefully the ideas and thoughts of women, and removing the causes of their turning away from men, is generally successful with them."

Chapter II About making acquaintance with the woman, and the efforts to win her over

Sutra 1 Ancient authors are of the opinion that a girl is not so easily seduced by a female messenger as by the efforts of the man himself, but that the wives of others are more easily got at through female messengers than by the personal efforts of the man.

Sutra 2 But Vatsyayana lays it down that whenever possible a man should act himself in these matters, and it is only when this is impracticable, or impossible, that female messengers should be used.

Sutra 3 There is a saying that women who act and talk boldly and freely are to be won by the man's personal efforts, and that women who do not possess those qualities are to be got at by female messengers.

Sutra 4 When a man acts for himself in the matter he should first of all make the acquaintance of the woman he loves in the following manner:

Sutras 5–6 He should arrange to be seen by the woman, either on a natural or special opportunity. A natural opportunity is when one of them goes to the house of the other, and a special opportunity is when they meet at the house of a friend, a kinsman, a minister or a physician, as also on the occasion of marriage ceremonies, sacrifices, festivals, funerals and garden parties.

Sutra 7 When they do meet, the man should be careful to look at the woman in such a way as to cause his state of mind to be made known to her; he should pull about his moustache, make a sound with his nails, cause his own ornaments to tinkle, bite his lower lip, and make various other signs of that description. When she is looking at him he should speak to his friends about her and other women, and should show to her his liberality and his appreciation of enjoyments. When sitting by the side of a female friend he should yawn and twist his body, contract his eyebrows, speak very slowly as if he was weary, and listen to her indifferently. A conversation having two meanings should also be carried on with a child or some other person, apparently having regard to a third person, but really having reference to the woman he loves, and in this way his love should be made manifest under the pretext of referring to others rather than to her. He should make marks that refer to her, on the earth with his nails, or with a stick, and should embrace and kiss a child in her presence, and give it the mixture of betel nut and leaves with his tongue, and press its chin with his fingers in a caressing way. All these things should be done at the proper time and in proper places.

Sutra 8 The man should fondle a child that may be sitting on her lap, and give it something to play with, and also take the same back again. Conversation with respect to the child may also be held with her, and in this manner he should gradually become well acquainted with her, and he should also make himself agreeable to her relations. Afterwards, this acquaintance should be made a pretext for visiting her house frequently, and on such occasions he should converse on the subject of love in her absence but within her hearing.

Sutra 9 As his intimacy with her increases he should leave some belongings with her on trust, and take them back a small portion at a time.

Sutra 10 Or he may give her some fragrant substances or betel nuts to be kept for him by her.

Sutra 11 After this he should endeavour to make her well acquainted with his own wife, and get them to carry on confidential conversations and to sit together in lonely places.

Sutra 12 In order to see her frequently he should arrange it so that the same goldsmith, the same jeweler, the same basketmaker, the same dyer and the same washerman should be employed by the two families.

Sutra 13 And he should also pay her long visits openly under the pretence of being engaged with her on business, and one business should lead to another, so as to keep up the intercourse between them.

Sura 14 Whenever she wants anything, or is in need of money, or wishes to acquire skill in one of the arts, he should give her to understand that he is willing and able to do anything that she wants, to give her money, or teach her one of the arts – all these things being quite within his ability and power.

Sutra 15 In the same way, he should hold discussions with her in company with other people, and they should talk of the doings and sayings of other persons, and examine different things, like jewelry, precious stones, and so on.

Sutra 16 On such occasions he should show her certain things, the

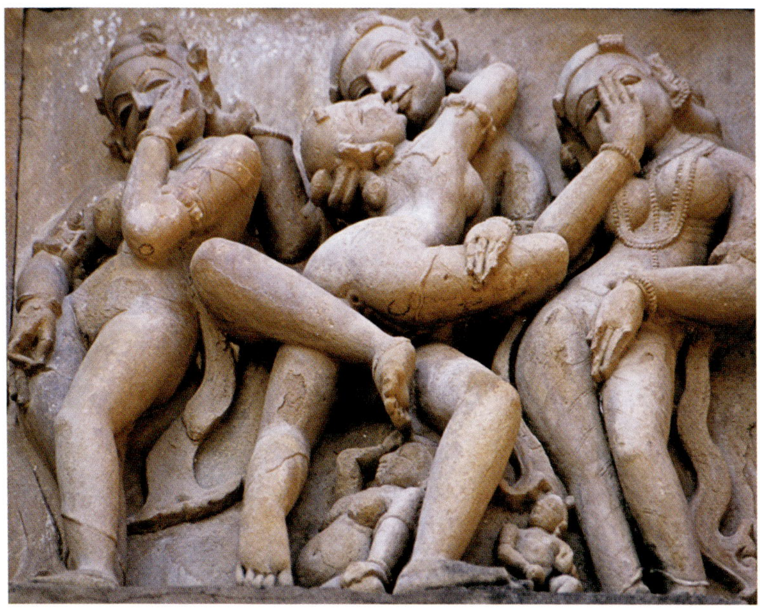

values of which she may be unacquainted with, and if she begins to dispute with him about the things or their value he should not contradict her, but point out that he agrees with her in every way.

Thus ends the ways of making the acquaintance of a woman.

Sutra 17 Now after a girl has become acquainted with the man as above described, and has manifested her love to him by the various outward signs and by the motions of her body, the man should make every effort to gain her over.

Sutra 18 But as girls are not acquainted with sexual union, they should be treated with the greatest delicacy, and the man should proceed with considerable caution.

Sutra 19 In the case of other women, accustomed to sexual intercourse, this caution is not necessary.

Sutra 20 When the intentions of the girl are known, and her bashfulness put aside, the man should begin to make use of her money, and an interchange of clothes or flowers should be made.

Sutra 21 In this matter the man should take particular care that the things given by him are handsome and valuable. Moreover, he should receive from her a mixture of betel nut and betel leaves, and when he is going to a party he should ask for the flower in her hair, or for the flower in her hand.

Sutra 22 If he himself gives her a flower it should be a sweet-smelling one, and should bear marks made by his nails or teeth.

Sutra 23 With a gradual approach he should dispel her fears, and by degrees get her to go with him to some lonely place, and there he should embrace and kiss her.

Sutra 24 And finally, at the time of giving her some betel nut, or of receiving the same from her, or at the time of making an exchange of flowers, he should touch and press her private parts, thus bringing his efforts to a satisfactory conclusion.

Sutra 25 When a man is endeavouring to seduce one woman, he should not attempt to seduce any other at the same time. But after he has succeeded with the first, and enjoyed her for a considerable time, he can keep her affections by giving her presents that she likes, and then commence making up to another woman.

Sutra 26 When a man sees the husband of a woman going to some place near his house, he should not enjoy the woman then, even though she may be easily won over at that time.

Sutra 27 A wise man having a regard for his reputation should not think of seducing a woman who is apprehensive, timid, not to be trusted, well guarded, or possessed of a father-in-law or mother-in-law.

Chapter III Examination of the state of a woman's mind

Sutras 1–2 When a man is trying to win over a woman he should examine the state of her mind and act as follows:

If she listens to him, but does not reveal to him in any way her own intentions, he should then try to win her over by means of a go-between.

Sutras 3–4 If she meets him once, and comes to meet him again but better dressed than before, or comes to him in some lonely place, he can be certain that she may be enjoyed through the use of a little force.

Sutras 5–6 A woman who lets a man make up to her, but does not give herself up, even after a long time, should be considered as a trifler in love, but owing to the fickleness of the human mind, even such a woman can be conquered by always keeping up a close acquaintance with her.

Sutra 7 When a woman avoids the attentions of a man, and on account of respect for him, and pride in herself, will not meet him or approach him, she can be won over only with difficulty, either by endeavouring to keep on familiar terms with her, or else by an exceedingly clever go-between.

Sutra 8 When a man makes an advance to a woman and she reproaches him with harsh words, she should be abandoned at once.

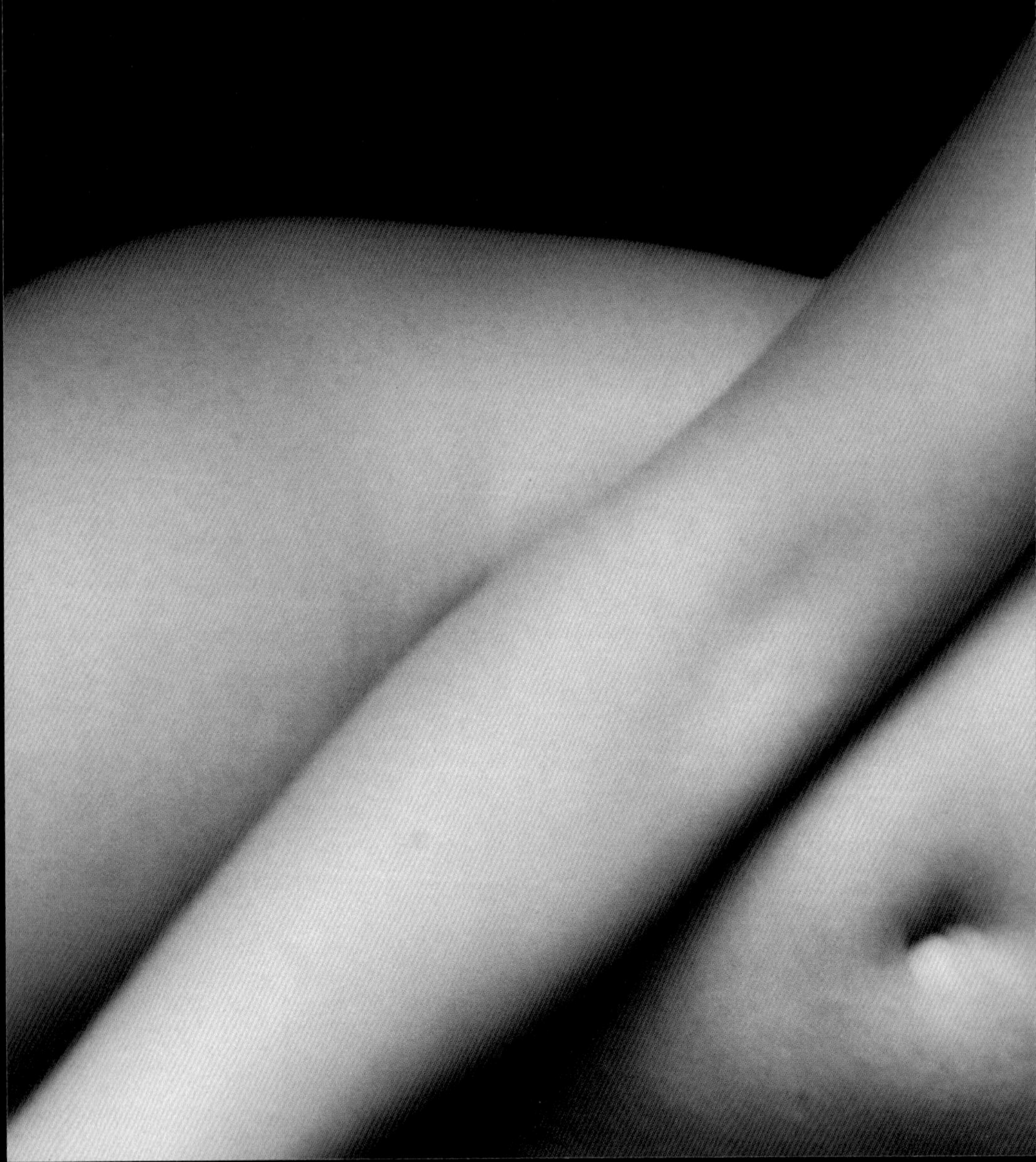

Sutra 9 When a woman reproaches a man, but at the same time acts affectionately toward him, she should be made love to in every way.

Sutra 10 A woman who meets a man in secluded places and puts up with the touch of his foot, but pretends, on account of the indecision of her mind, not to be aware of it should be conquered by patience, and by continuous efforts as follows:

Sutra 11 If she happens to go to sleep in his vicinity he should put his left arm round her, and see when she awakes whether she rebuffs him in reality, or only rebuffs him in such a way as if she desired the same thing be done to her again.

Sutra 12 And what is done by the arm can also be done by the foot.

Sutra 13 If the man succeeds in this point he should embrace her more closely.

Sutra 14 And if she will not stand the embrace and gets up, but behaves with him as usual the next day, he should consider then that she is not unwilling to be enjoyed by him.

Sutra 15 If, however, she does not appear again, the man should try to get over her by means of a go-between; and if, after having disappeared for some time, she again appears, and behaves with him as usual, the man should then consider that she would not object to being united with him.

Sutra 16 When a woman gives a man an opportunity, and makes her own interest in him apparent, he should proceed to enjoy her. And the signs of a woman demonstrating her love are these:

Sutra 17 She calls out to a man without being addressed by him in the first instance.

Sutra 18 She shows herself to him in lonely places.

Sutra 19 She trembles and is inarticulate when talking to him.

Sutra 20 The fingers of her hand, and the toes of her feet, become moistened with perspiration and her face blooms with delight.

Sutra 21 She shampoos his body and presses his head.

Sutra 22 When shampooing him she works with one hand only, and with the other she touches and embraces parts of his body.

Sutra 23 She remains motionless with both hands placed on his body, as if she had been surprised by something, or was overcome by fatigue.

Sutra 24 She sometimes rests her face upon his thighs, and when asked to shampoo them does not show any unwillingness to do so.

Sutra 25 She places one of her hands quite motionless on his body, and even though the man presses it between two parts of his body, she does not remove it for a long time.

Sutra 26 Lastly, when she has resisted all the efforts of the man to win her over, she returns to him the next day to shampoo his body as before.

Sutras 27–30 When a woman neither gives encouragement to a man nor avoids him, but hides herself and remains in some lonely place, she must be got at by means of the female servant who may be near her. If when called by the man she acts in the same way, then she should be won over by means of a skilful go-between. But if she has nothing to say to the man, he should think carefully before he begins any further attempts to win her over.

Thus ends the examination of the state of a woman's mind.

Sutra 31 A man should first get himself introduced to a woman, and then carry on a conversation with her. He should give her hints of his love for her, and if he finds from her replies that she receives these hints favourably, he should then set to work without any fear to win her over.

Sutra 32 A woman who shows her love by outward signs to the man at his first interview should be won over very easily.

Sutra 33 In the same way, a lascivious woman who, when addressed in loving words, replies openly in words that express her love should, at that very moment, be considered to have been won over. With regard to all women, whether they be wise, simple or confiding, this rule is laid down that those who manifest their love openly are easily won over.

Chapter IV About the business of a go-between

Sutra 1 If a woman has manifested her love or desire, either by signs or by motions of the body, and is afterwards rarely or never seen anywhere, or if a woman is met for the first time, the man should get a go-between to approach her.

Sutra 2 Now the go-between, having wheedled herself into the confidence of the woman by acting according to her disposition, should try to make her hate or despise her husband by holding artful conversations with her, by telling her about medicines for getting children, by talking to her about other people, by tales of various kinds, by stories about the wives of other men, and by praising her beauty, wisdom, generosity and good nature.

Sutras 3–4 And then say to her: "It is indeed a pity that you, who are so excellent a woman in every way, should be possessed of a husband of this kind. Beautiful lady, he is not fit even to serve you."

Sutra 5 The go-between should talk further to the woman about the weakness of the passion of her husband, his jealousy, his roguery, his ingratitude, his aversion to enjoyments, his dullness, his meanness, and all the other faults that he may have and with which she may be acquainted.

Sutra 6 She should particularly harp upon that fault or that failing by which the wife may appear to be the most affected.

Sutra 7 If the wife be a deer woman, and the husband a hare man, then there would be no fault in that direction.

Sutra 8 But in the event of his being a hare man, and she being a mare woman or elephant woman, then this fault should be pointed out to her.

Sutra 9 Gonikaputra is of the opinion that when it is the first affair of the woman, or when her love has been shown only very secretly, the man should then secure and send to her a go-between, with whom she may be already acquainted, and in whom she confides.

Sutras 10–11 But to return to our subject. The go-between should tell the woman about the obedience and love of the man, and as her

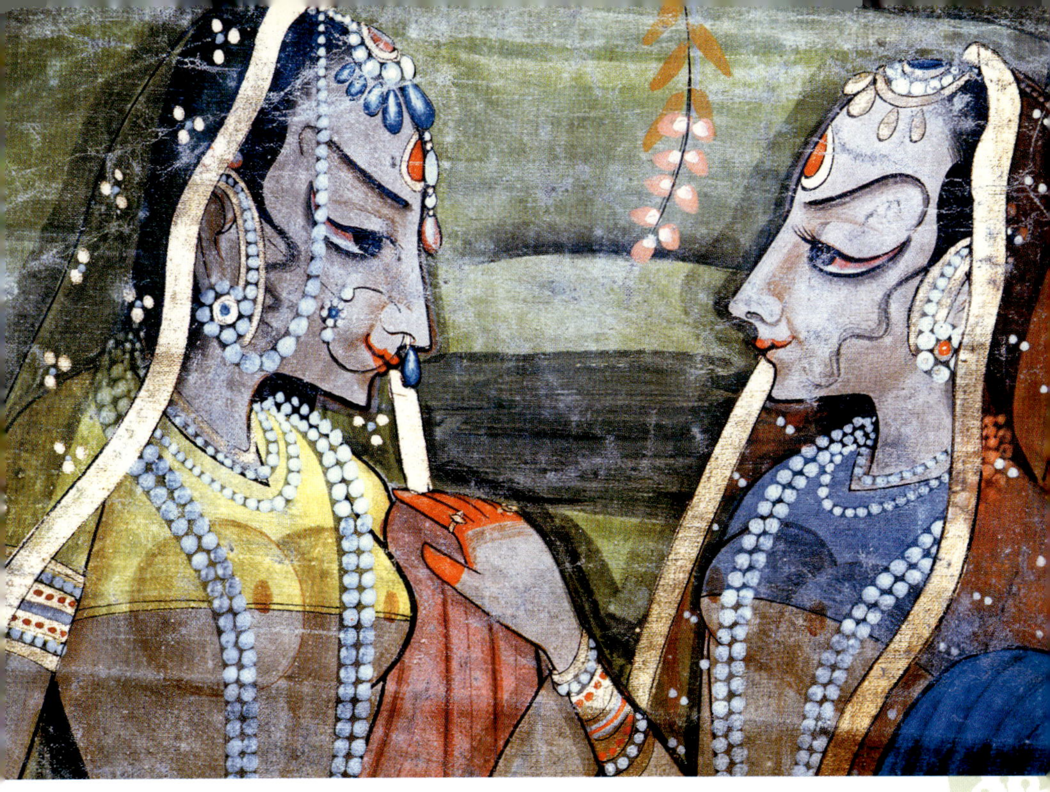

confidence and affection increase, she should then explain to her the thing to be accomplished in the following way.

Sutra 12 "Hear this, oh beautiful lady, that this man, born of a good family, having seen you, has gone mad on your account. The poor young man, who is tender by nature, has never been distressed in such a way before, and it is highly probable that he will succumb under his present affliction and experience the pains of death."

Sutra 13 If the woman listens with a favourable ear, then on the following day the go-between, having observed signs of good spirits in her face, in her eyes and in her manner of conversation, should again converse with her on the subject of the man.

Sutra 14 The go-between should tell her the stories of Ahalya[1] and Indra, of Sakuntala[2] and Dushyanta, and such others as may befit the occasion.

Sutra 15 She should also describe to her the strength of the man, his talents, his skill in the sixty-four sorts of enjoyments mentioned by Babhravya, his good looks, and his liaison with some praiseworthy woman, no matter whether this last ever took place or not.

Sutra 16 In addition to this, the go-between should carefully note the behaviour of the woman, which if favourable would be as follows:

Sutras 17–18 She would address her with a smile, would seat herself close beside her, and ask her, "Where have you been? What have you been doing? Where did you dine? Where did you sleep? Where have you been sitting?"

Sutras 19–21 Moreover, the woman would meet the go-between in a lonely place and tell her anecdotes there, would yawn contemplatively and heave long sighs of desire.

Sutras 22–24 She would give her presents, remember her at the times of festivals and dismiss her with a wish to see her again.

Sutras 25–26 She would say to her jestingly, "Oh, well-speaking woman, why do you speak these bad words to me?", and then would discourse on the sin of her union with the man.

Sutras 27–28 She would not tell her about any previous visits or conversations that she may have had with him, but wish to be asked about these, and lastly would laugh at the man's desire, but would not reproach him in any way.

Thus ends the behaviour of the woman with the go-between.

Sutras 29–30 When the woman manifests her love in the manner above described, the go-between should increase it by bringing to her love tokens from the man. But if the woman is not acquainted with the man personally, the go-between should win her over by extolling and praising his good qualities, and by telling stories about his love for her.

Sutra 31 Here Auddalaka says that when a man and woman are not personally acquainted with each other, and have not shown each other any signs of affection, the employment of a go-between is useless.

Sutra 32 The followers of Babhravya on the other hand affirm that even though they be personally unacquainted, provided they have shown each other signs of affection a go-between can be employed.

Sutra 33 Gonikaputra asserts that a go-between should be employed, provided they are acquainted with each other, even though no signs of affection may have passed between them.

Sutra 34 Vatsyayana, however, lays it down that even though they may not be personally acquainted with each other, and may not have shown each other any signs of affection, still they are both capable of placing confidence in a go-between.

Sutra 35 Now the go-between should show the woman the presents, such as the betel nut and betel leaves, the perfumes, the flowers and the rings that the man may have given to her for the sake of the woman.

Sutra 36 And on these presents the marks of the man's teeth and nails, and other signs, should be impressed.

Sutra 37 On the cloth that he may send he should draw with saffron both his hands joined together as if in earnest entreaty.

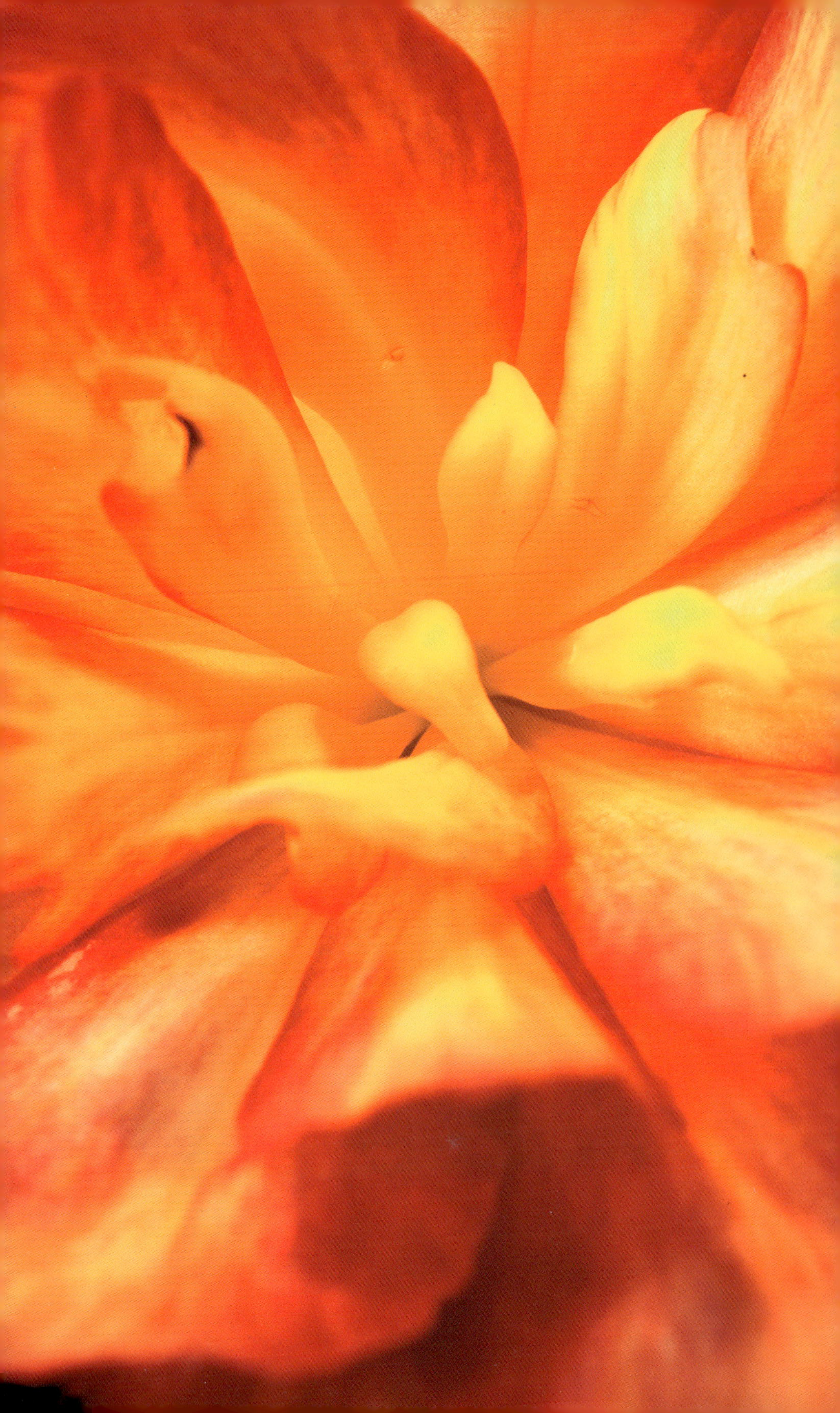

Sutra 38 The go-between should also show to the woman ornamental figures of various kinds cut in leaves, together with ear ornaments, and chaplets made of flowers containing love letters expressing the desire of the man.

Sutra 39 She should encourage her to send him presents in return.

Sutra 40 After they have mutually accepted each other's presents, then a meeting should be arranged between them on the faith of the go-between.

Sutra 41 The followers of Babhravya say that this meeting should take place when going to a temple, or during an occasion such as a fair, garden party, theatrical performance, marriage, sacrifice, festival or funeral; it could also be when going to the river to bathe, or at a time of natural calamity, when fearing robbers or an invasion of the country.

Sutra 42 Gonikaputra is of the opinion that these meetings are better brought about in the abodes of female friends, mendicants, astrologers and ascetics.

Sutra 43 But Vatsyayana believes that a place is only well suited for the purpose if it has an appropriate means of entry and exit, and where arrangements have been made to prevent any accidental occurrence, and when a man who has once entered the house can also leave it at the proper time without any disagreeable encounter.

Sutra 44 Go-betweens or female messengers are of the following different kinds:

A go-between who takes upon herself the whole burden of the business

A go-between who does only a limited part of the business
A go-between who is the bearer of a letter or message only
A go-between acting for herself
The go-between of an innocent young woman
A wife serving as a go-between
A silent go-between
A go-between who "acts the part of the wind"

Sutras 45–48 A woman who, having observed the mutual passion of a man and woman, brings them together and arranges it by the power of her own intellect, such a one is called a go-between who takes upon herself the whole burden of the business. This kind of go-between is chiefly employed when the man and the woman are already acquainted with each other, and have conversed together, and in such cases she is sent not only by the man (as is always done in all other cases) but also by the woman. The above name is also given to a go-between who, perceiving that the man and the woman are suited to each other, tries to bring about a union between them, even though they are not acquainted with each other.

Sutras 49–51 A go-between who, perceiving that some part of the affair is already done or that the advances on the part of the man have already been made, completes the rest of the business is called a go-between who performs only a limited part of the business.

A go-between who simply carries messages between a man and a woman who love each other but who cannot meet frequently is called the bearer of a letter or message.

Sutra 52 This name is also given to one who is sent by either of the lovers to acquaint either the one or the other with the time and place of their meeting.

Sutra 53 A woman who goes herself to a man, and tells him of a dream she has had in which she has enjoyed sexual union with him. She expresses her anger at his wife – who has rebuked him after he called his wife by the name of her rival instead of by her own name – and gives him something bearing the marks of her teeth and nails, and informs him that she knew she was formerly desired by him, and asks him privately whether she or his wife is the better looking. Such a person is called a woman who is a go-between for herself. Now such a woman should be met and interviewed by the man in private and secretly.

Sutras 54–55 The above name is also given to a woman who having been asked by some other woman to act as her go-between then wins over the man to herself by making him personally acquainted with herself and thus causes the other woman to fail.

Sutra 56 The same applies to a man who, acting as a go-between for another, and having no previous connection with the woman, wins her for himself and thus causes the failure of the other man.

Sutra 57 A woman who has gained the confidence of the innocent young wife of any man, and who has learned her secrets without exercising any pressure on her mind, and found out from her how her husband behaves to her, if this woman then teaches her the art of securing his favour, and decorates her so as to show her love, and instructs her how and when to be angry, or to pretend to be so, and then, having herself made marks of the nails and teeth on the body of the wife, gets the latter to send for her husband to show these marks to him, and thus excite him for enjoyment, such is called the go-between of an innocent young woman.

Sutra 58 In such cases the man should reply through the same woman.

Sutra 59 When a man gets his wife to gain the confidence of a woman whom he wants to enjoy, and to call on her and talk to her about the wisdom and ability of her husband, that wife is called a wife serving as a go-between. In this case the feelings of the woman for the man should also be made known through the wife.

Sutra 60 When any man sends a girl or a female servant to any woman under some pretext or other, and places a letter in her bouquet of flowers, or in her ear ornaments, or marks something about her with his teeth or nails, that girl or female servant is called a silent go-between. In this case the man should expect an answer from the woman through the same person.

Sutra 61 A person who carries a message to a woman which has a double meaning, or which relates to some past transactions, or which is unintelligible to other people, is called a go-between who "acts the part of the wind". In this case the reply should be asked for through the same woman.

Thus ends discussion of the different kinds of go-between.

Sutra 62 A female astrologer, a female servant, a female beggar and a female artist are well acquainted with the business of a go-between, and very soon gain the confidence of other women.

Sutra 63 Any one of them can raise enmity between any two persons if she wishes to do so, or can extol the loveliness of any woman that she wishes to praise, or can describe the arts practised by other women in sexual union.

Sutra 64 They can also speak highly of the love of a man, of his skill in sexual enjoyment, and of the desire of other women – more beautiful

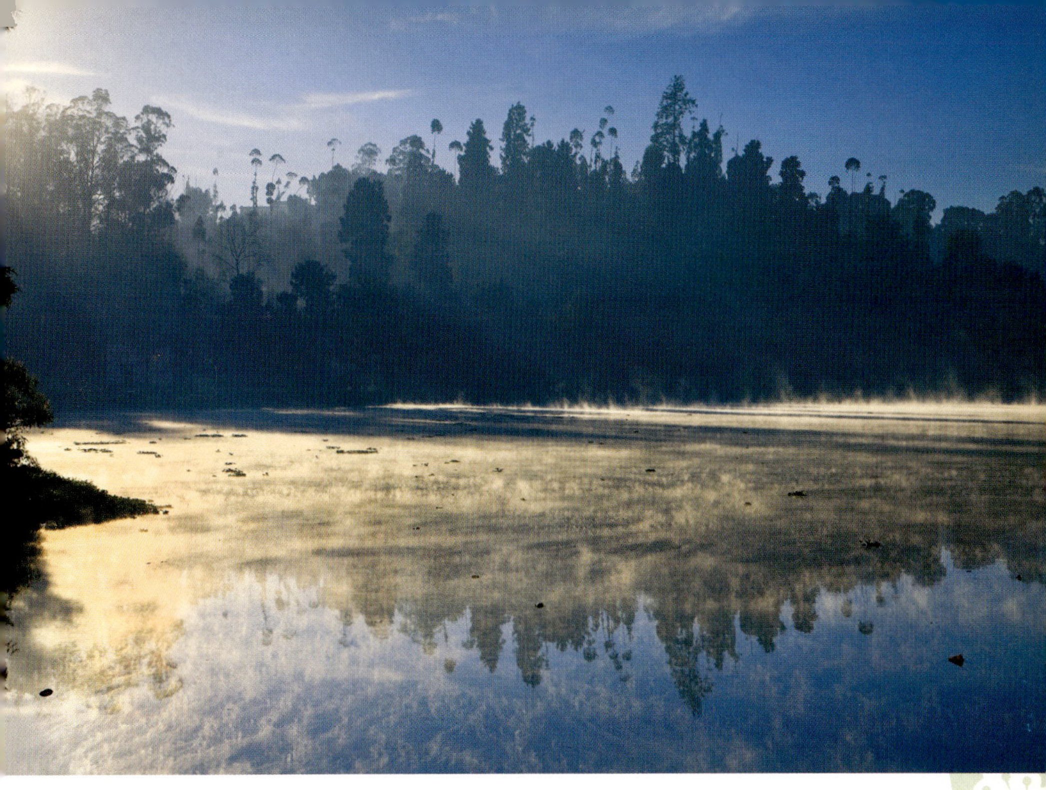

even than the woman they are addressing – for him, and explain the restraint under which he may be at home.

Sutra 65 Lastly, a go-between can, by the artfulness of her conversation, unite a woman with a man even though he may not have been thought of by her, or may have been considered beyond her aspirations. She can also bring back a man to a woman, who, owing to some cause or other, has separated himself from her.

Chapter V About the love of persons in authority for the wives of other men

Sutras 1–2 Kings and their ministers have no access to the abodes of others, and moreover their mode of living is constantly watched and observed and imitated by the people at large, just as animals seeing the sun rise, get up after that, and when it sets in the evening, lies down again.

Sutras 3–4 Persons in authority should not therefore do any improper act in public, because such are impossible from their position and would be deserving of censure. But if they find that such an act is necessary, they should make use of the proper means as described in the following paragraphs.

Sutra 5 The head man of the village, the king's officer employed there, and the man whose business it is to glean corn, can win over female villagers simply by asking them. It is on this account that women of this class are called unchaste by those devoted to sensual pleasure.

Sutra 6 The union of the above-mentioned men with this class of woman takes place when they are engaged in unpaid labour, when filling the granaries in their houses, when taking things in and out of the house, when cleaning the house, when working in the fields, and when purchasing cotton, wool, flax, hemp and thread, and during the season of the purchase, sale and exchange of various other articles, as well as when doing various other work.

Sutra 7 In the same way the superintendents of cowpens enjoy the women in the cowpens.

Sutra 8 And yarn officers have their way with widows, women who have left their husbands and destitute women.

Sutra 9 The intelligent accomplish their object by wandering at night in the village, which is when villagers unite with their daughters-in-law, being much alone with them.

Sutra 10 Lastly, the superintendents of markets have a great deal to do with the female villagers when they make purchases in the market.

Sutra 11 During the festival of the eighth moon – that is, during the bright half of the month of Margashirsha [22 November–21 December] – and during the moonlight festival of the month of Kartika [23 October–21 November], and the spring festival of Chaitra [the beginning of the Hindu New Year], the women of cities and towns generally visit the women of the king's harem in the royal palace.

Sutra 12 These visitors go to the various apartments of the women of the harem, as they are acquainted with them, and pass the night in conversation with them, and in proper sports and amusement, then depart early the next morning.

Sutras 13–14 On such occasions a female attendant of the king (previously acquainted with the woman whom the king desires) should loiter, accost the woman when she sets out to go home and induce her to come and see beautiful things in the palace.

Sutras 15–16 Prior to these festivals the female attendant should have intimated to the woman that on the occasion of this festival she would show her all the beautiful things in the royal palace.

Sutra 17 Accordingly, she should show her the bower of the coral creeper, the garden house with its floor inlaid with precious stones, the bower of grapes, the building on the water, the secret passages in the walls of the palace, the pictures, the sporting animals, the machines, the birds, and the cages of the lions and the tigers.

Sutras 18–20 After this, when alone with her, she should tell her about the king's love for her, and should describe to her the good fortune which would attend upon her union with the king, giving her a strict promise of secrecy.

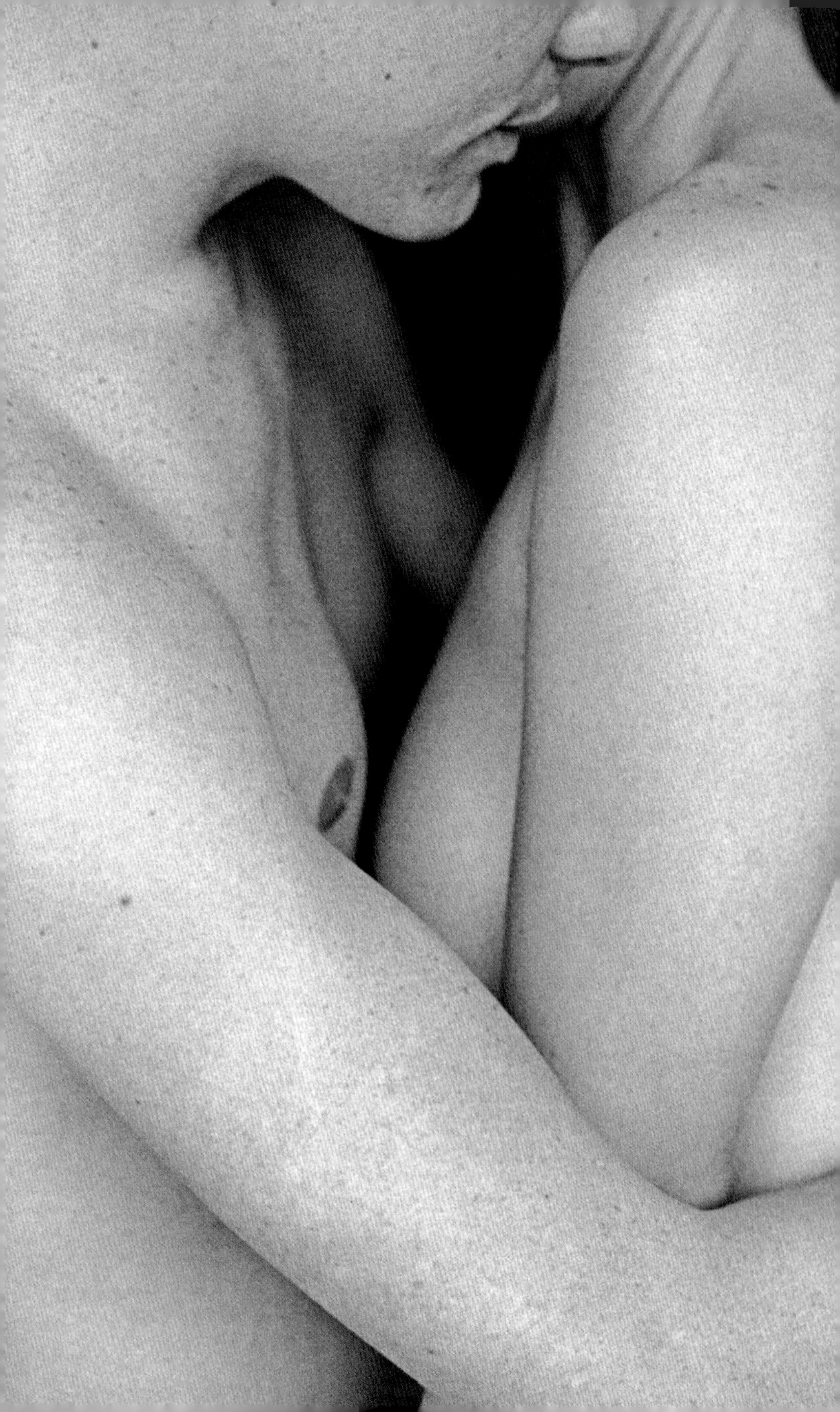

Sutra 21 If the woman does not accept the offer, she should conciliate and please her with handsome presents befitting the position of the king, and having accompanied her for some distance she should dismiss her with great affection.

Sutra 22 Or, having made the acquaintance of the husband of the woman whom the king desires, the wives of the king should get the wife to pay them a visit in the harem, and on this occasion a female attendant of the king, having been sent thither, should act as above described.

Sutra 23 Or, one of the king's wives should get acquainted with the woman that the king desires, by sending one of the female attendants to her, who should, on their becoming more intimate, induce her to come and see the royal abode. Afterwards, when she has visited the harem and acquired confidence, a female confidante of the king should be sent there to act as described earlier.

Sutra 24 Or, the king's wife should invite the woman the king desires to come to the royal palace so that she might see the king's wife practise an art in which she is skilled, and after the woman has come to the harem, a female attendant of the king should be sent there to act as described earlier.

Sutra 25 Or, a female beggar, acting in league with the king's wife, should say to the woman desired by the king, and whose husband may have lost his wealth or may have some reason to fear the king: "This wife of the king has influence over him, and she is, moreover, naturally kind-hearted, we must therefore go to her about this matter. I shall arrange for your entrance into the harem, and she will do away with all cause of danger and fear from the king." If the woman accepts this offer, the female beggar should take her two or three times to the harem, and the king's wife there should promise her protection. After this, when the woman – delighted with her reception and the promise of protection – again goes to the harem, a female attendant of the king should be sent there to act as described earlier.

Sutra 26 What has been said above regarding the wife of one who has some reason to fear the king applies also to the wives of those who seek service under the king, or who are oppressed by the king's ministers, or who are poor, or who are not satisfied with their position, or who desire to gain the king's favour, or who wish to become famous among the people, or who are oppressed by the members of their own caste, or who want to injure their caste fellows, or who are spies of the king, or who have any other object to attain.

Sutra 27 Lastly, if the woman desired by the king is living with some person who is not her husband, then the king will have her arrested, and, having made her a slave on account of her crime, he will place her in the harem.

Sutra 28 Or the king should cause his ambassador to quarrel with the husband of the woman he desires, and should then imprison her as the wife of an enemy, and by this means should place her in the harem.

Thus ends the discussion of the means of winning over the wives of others secretly.

Sutra 29 The above-mentioned ways of winning over the wives of other men are practised chiefly in the palaces of kings. But a king should never enter the abode of another person.

Sutra 30 Abhira, the king of the Kottas, was killed by a washerman while in the house of another, and in the same way Jayasana, the king of the Kashis, was slain by the commander of his cavalry.

Sutra 31 But according to the customs of some countries there are unimpeded opportunities for kings to make love to other men's wives.

Sutra 32 Thus in the country of the Andhras[3] the newly married daughters of the people enter the king's harem with some presents on the tenth day of their marriage, and having been enjoyed by the king they are then dismissed.

Sutra 33 In the country of the Vatsagulmas[4] the wives of the chief ministers approach the king at night to serve him.

Sutra 34 In the country of the Vaidarbhas[5] the beautiful wives of the inhabitants pass a month in the king's harem under the pretence of affection for the king.

Sutra 35 In the country of the Aparatakas[6] the people give their beautiful wives as presents to the ministers and the kings.

Sutra 36 And, lastly, in the country of the Saurashtras[7] the women of the city and the country enter the royal harem for the king's pleasure, either in groups or separately.

There are also two verses on the subject as follows:

Sutra 37 "These are the various means and ways used by different kings in different places with regard to the wives of other persons."

Sutra 38 "But a king who has the welfare of his people at heart should not on any account put these various means and ways into practice."

"A king who has conquered the six[8] enemies of mankind becomes the master of the whole earth."

Chapter VI About the women of the royal harem; and of the keeping of one's own wife

Sutra 1 The women of the royal harem cannot see or meet any men on account of their being strictly guarded, neither do they have their desires satisfied because their only husband is common to many wives. For this reason among themselves they give pleasure to each other in various ways as now described.

Sutras 2–3 Having dressed the daughters of their nurses, their female friends or female attendants like men, they accomplish their object by means of bulbs, roots and fruits which have the form of the *lingam*, or they lie down upon the statue of a male figure with the *lingam* visible and erect.

Sutra 4 Some kings, who are compassionate, take or apply certain medicines to enable them to enjoy many wives in one night, simply for the purpose of satisfying the desire of their women, though they perhaps have no desire of their own. Others enjoy with great affection only those wives whom they particularly like, while others take each wife according to her turn as it arrives in due course. Such are the customs prevalent in the East.

Sutra 5 What is said about the means of enjoyment of the female is also applicable to the male.

Sutra 6 By means of their female attendants the ladies of the royal harem generally get men into their apartments disguised as women.

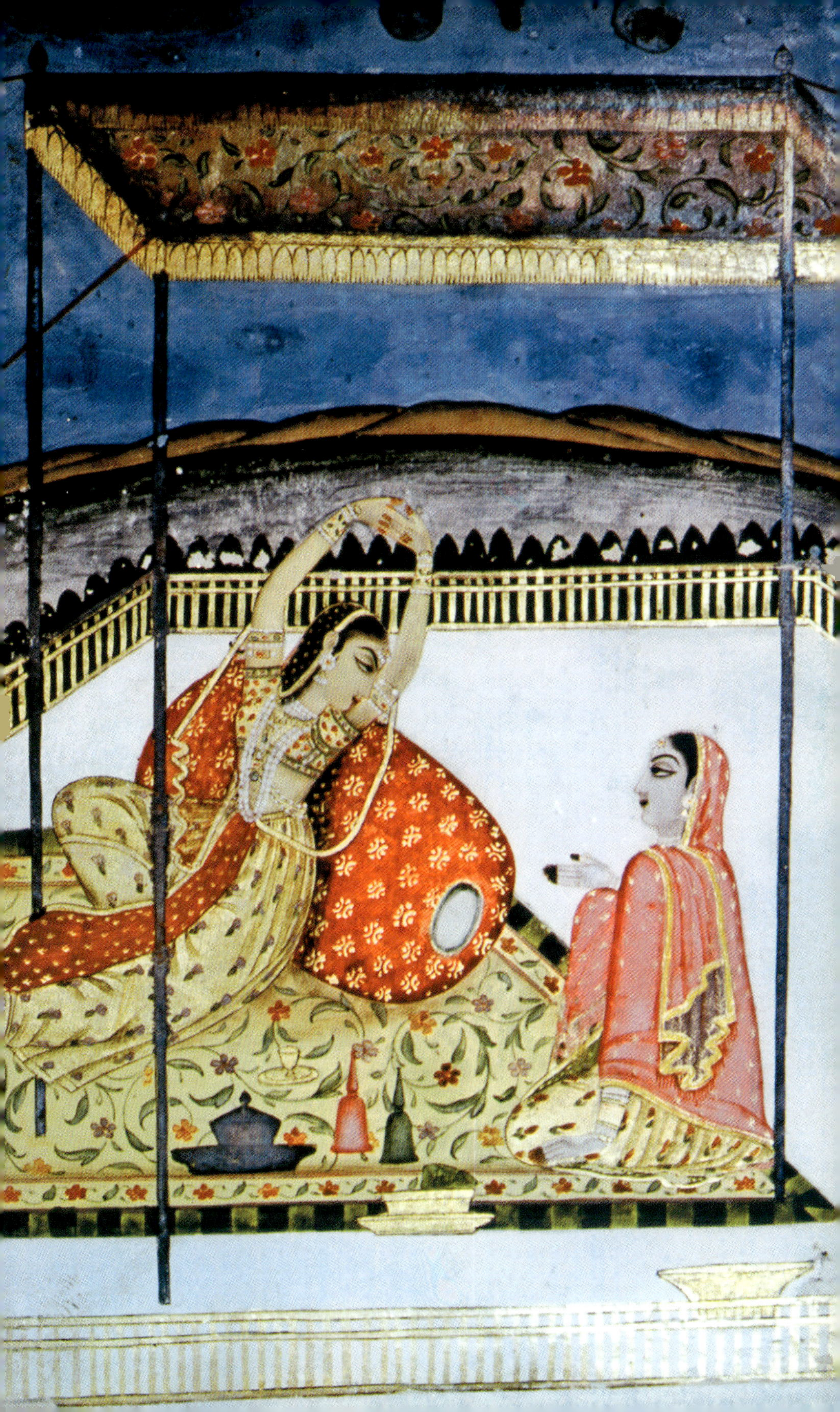

Sutra 7 Their female attendants, and the daughters of their nurses, who are acquainted with the secret desires of the women in the harem, should try to get men to come to the harem by telling them of the good fortune awaiting them.

Sutra 8 They should convey relevant information such as how to enter and leave the palace, the size of the premises, the degree of vigilance of the guards, and the carelessness and irregularities of those attending the royal wives.

Sutra 9 But these women should never induce a man to enter the harem by telling him falsehoods, for that would probably endanger his safety.

Sutra 10 As for the man himself, he had better not enter a royal harem, even though it may be easily accessible, on account of the numerous dangers to which he may be exposed there.

Sutras 11–13 If, however, he wants to enter it, he should first ascertain whether there is an easy way to get out, whether it is closely surrounded by the pleasure garden, whether it has separate enclosures belonging to it, whether the guards are careless, whether the king has gone abroad – and then, when he is called by the women of the harem, he should carefully observe the area and enter by the way that they have pointed out. If he is able to manage it, he should hang about the harem every day, and under some pretext or other make friends with the guards.

Sutra 14 He should show himself attached to a female attendant of the harem, who may have become acquainted with his design, and to whom he should express his regret at not being able to obtain the object of his desire.

Sutra 15 Lastly, he should cause the whole business of a go-between to be done by the woman who may have access to the harem.

Sutra 16 He should be careful to recognize the emissaries of the king.

Sutras 17–18 When a go-between has no access to the harem, then the man should stand in some place where the lady whom he loves and whom he is anxious to enjoy can be seen. If that place is occupied by the king's guards, he should then disguise himself as a female attendant of the lady who comes to the place, or passes by it.

Sutra 19 When she looks at him he should let her know his feelings by outward signs and gestures.

Sutra 20 And he should show her pictures, things with double meanings, chaplets of flowers and rings.

Sutra 21 He should carefully mark the answer she gives, whether by word, sign or gesture, and he should then try to get into the harem.

Sutra 22 If he is certain of her coming to some particular place he should conceal himself there.

Sutras 23–24 At the appointed time he should enter along with her as one of the guards.

He may also go in and out, concealed in a folded bed, or blanket.

Sutra 25 Or he can make his body invisible[9] by means of external applications.

Sutra 26 A recipe for one of these is as follows: the heart of a

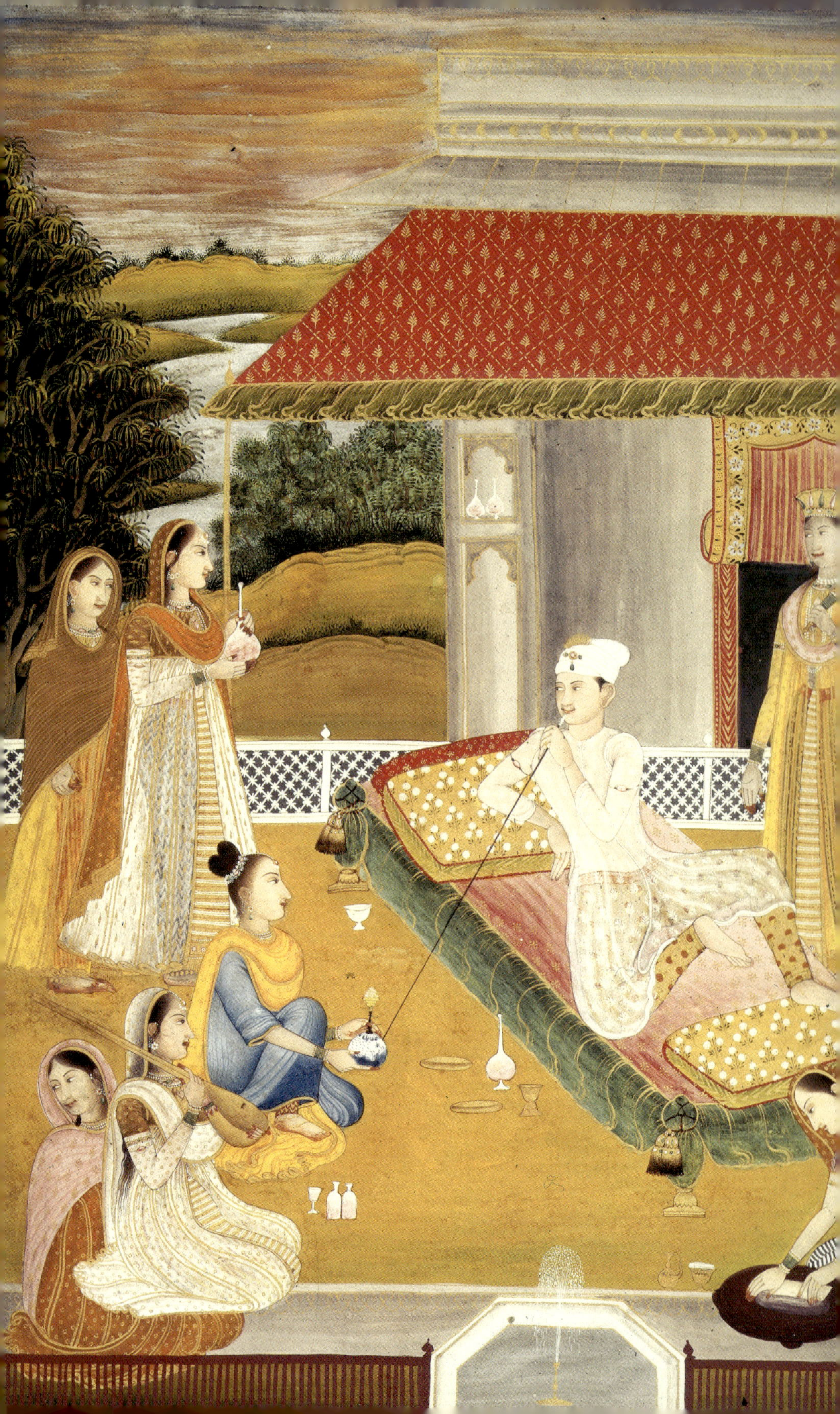

mongoose, the fruit of the long gourd (*tumbi*) and the eyes of a serpent should all be burned without letting out the smoke. The ashes should then be ground and mixed with an equal amount of water. By putting this mixture upon his eyes a man can go about unseen.

Sutra 27 Again the man may enter the harem during the festival of the eighth moon in the month of Margashirsha, and during the moonlight festivals when the female attendants of the harem are all busily occupied, or in confusion.

The following principles are laid down on this subject.

Sutras 28–30 The entry of young men into harems, and their exit from them, generally take place when things are being brought into the palace, or when things are being taken out of it, or when drinking festivals are going on, or when the female attendants are in a hurry, or when the residence of some of the royal ladies is being changed, or when the king's wives go to gardens, or to fairs, or when they enter the palace on their return from them, or, lastly, when the king is absent on a long pilgrimage.

Sutras 31–32 The women of the royal harem know each other's secrets, and having but one object to attain, they give assistance to each other. A young man, who enjoys all of them, and who is common to them all, can continue enjoying his union with them so long as it is kept quiet, and is not known abroad.

Sutra 33 Now in the country of the Aparatakas the royal ladies are not well protected, and consequently many young men are passed into the harem by those women who have access to the royal palace.

Sutra 34 The wives of the king of the Ahira country accomplish their objects with those guards in the harem who are Kshatriyas.

Sutra 35 The royal ladies in the country of the Vatsagulmas cause such men as are suitable to enter into the harem along with their female messengers.

Sutra 36 In the country of the Vaidarbhas the sons of the royal ladies enter the royal harem when they please and enjoy the women, with the exception of their own mothers.

Sutra 37 In the Strirajya the wives of the king are enjoyed by his caste-fellows and relations.

Sutra 38 In the Ganda country the royal wives are enjoyed by Brahmins, friends, servants and slaves.

Sutra 39 In the Samdhava country servants, foster children and other persons like them enjoy the women of the harem.

Sutra 40 In the country of the Haimavatas adventurous citizens bribe the guards and enter the harem.

Sutra 41 In the country of the Vanyas and the Kalmyas, Brahmins, with the knowledge of the king, enter the harem under the pretence of giving flowers to the ladies, and speak with them from behind a curtain, and from such conversation union subsequently takes place.

Sutra 42 Lastly, the women in the harem of the king of the Prachyas conceal one young man in the harem for every batch of nine or ten of the women.

Thus act the wives of others.

Sutra 43 For these reasons a man should guard his own wife. Ancient sages say that a king should select for guards in his harem such men as have had their freedom from carnal desires well tested.

Sutra 44 But such men, though free themselves from carnal desire, may through fear or avarice cause other persons to enter the harem.

Sutra 45 Therefore Gonikaputra says that kings should place such men in the harem as may have had their freedom from carnal desires, fears and avarice well tested.

Sutra 46 Lastly, Vatsyayana says that under the influence of Dharma[10] people might be admitted, and therefore men should be selected who are free from carnal desires, fear, avarice and Dharma.[11]

Sutra 47 The followers of Babhravya say that a man should let his wife associate with a young woman who would tell him the secrets of other people, and thus test his wife's chastity.

Sutra 48 But Vatsyayana says that because wicked people are always successful with women, a man should not cause his innocent wife to be corrupted by introducing her into the company of a deceitful woman.

Sutra 49 The following cause the destruction of a woman's chastity:

Always going into society, and sitting in company
Absence of restraint
The loose habits of her husband
Want of caution in her relations with other men
Continued and long absence of her husband
Living in a foreign country
Destruction of her love and feelings by her husband

The company of loose women
The jealousy of her husband

There are also the following verses on the subject:

Sutra 50 "A clever man, learned in the *shastras* and the ways of winning over the wives of other people, is never deceived in the case of his own wives."

Sutra 51 "No one, however, should make use of these ways for seducing the wives of others, because they do not always succeed, and, moreover, they often cause disasters, and the destruction of Dharma and Artha."

Sutra 52 "This book, which is intended for the good of the people, and to teach them the ways of guarding their own wives, should not be made use of merely for winning over the wives of others."

NOTES

1. Ahalya, the beautiful wife of the sage Gautama Maharishi, was seduced by Indra, the king of the gods, who appeared in the form of her husband.
2. The best-known heroine in Sanskrit literature, dramatized by Kalidasa, Sakuntala was married to Dushyanta, founder of the Paurava dynasty.
3. The country of Tailangam, to the south of Rajahmundry.
4. Supposed to be a tract of the country to the south of Malwa.
5. Now known by the name Berar, its capital was Kundapura, identified with modern Amravati.
6. Also called Aparantakas, being the northern and southern Concan.
7. The modern provinces of Kathiawar. Its capital was called Girinagara, or the modern Junagadh.
8. These are lust, anger, avarice, ignorance, pride and envy.
9. The way to make oneself invisible, the knowledge of the art of transmigration, or changing ourselves or others into any shape or form by the use of charms and spells, the power of being in two places at once, and other occult sciences, are referred to frequently in oriental literature.
10. This may be considered to mean religious influence and alludes to people who may be won over by that means.
11. Eunuchs do not appear to have been employed in the king's harem in those days, though they seem to have been employed for other purposes. [See page 51.]

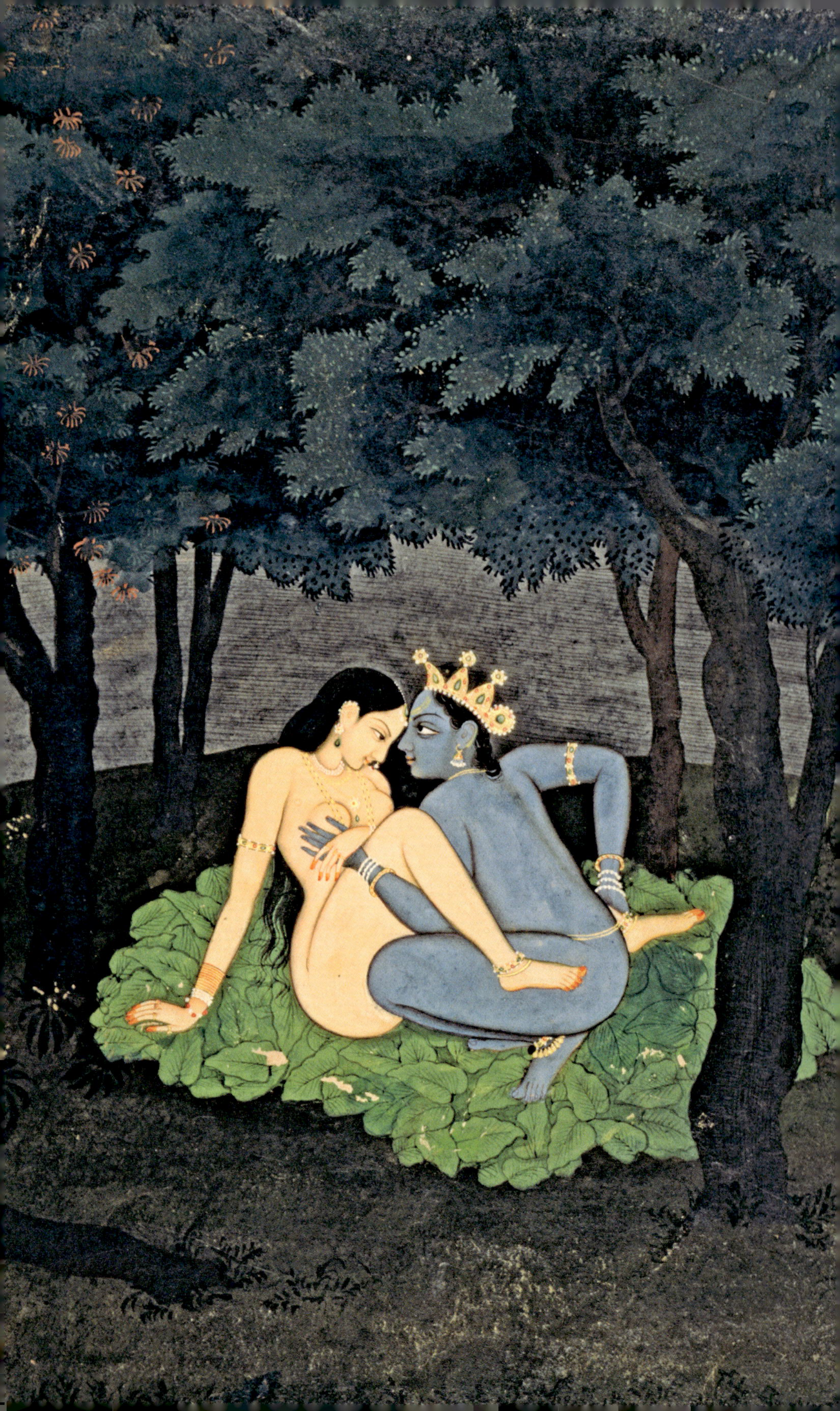

Part Six: On Courtesans and Their Way of Life

Introductory Remarks

This part, about courtesans, was prepared by Vatsyayana from a treatise written by Dattaka for the women of Pataliputra (modern Patna) some 2,000 years ago. Dattaka's work does not appear to be extant now, but this abridgement of it is quite equal to anything by Emile Zola and other naturalistic writers. Although a great deal has been written about the courtesan, a better description of her, her belongings, her ideas and the working of her mind than is contained in the following pages cannot be found anywhere.

A social history of early India would not be complete without mention of the courtesan. The Hindus had the good sense to recognize courtesans as a part of human society, who, provided they behaved themselves with decency and propriety, were even regarded with a certain respect. They have never been treated in the East with the contempt that is so common in the West, while their education has always been superior to that bestowed upon the rest of womankind in eastern countries.

In the early days the well-educated Hindu dancing girl and courtesan doubtless resembled the *hetera* of the Greeks, and, being educated and amusing, was a far more acceptable companion than most married or unmarried women of that period. At all times and in all countries there has always been some rivalry between the chaste and the unchaste. Although some women are born courtesans, and follow the instincts of their nature, it has been said by some that every woman has an inkling of the profession in her nature and does her best to make herself agreeable to the opposite sex.

The subtlety of women, their wonderful perceptive powers, their knowledge, and their intuitive appreciation of men and things are all shown in the following pages, which may be looked upon as a concentrated essence that has since been worked up into detail by many writers in every quarter of the globe.

Chapter I The causes of a courtesan resorting to men; the means of attaching to herself the man desired; and the kind of man that it is desirable to be acquainted with

Sutra 1 By having intercourse with men courtesans obtain sexual pleasure, as well as their own maintenance.

Sutras 2–3 Now when a courtesan takes up with a man from love, the action is natural; but when she resorts to him for the purpose of getting money, her action is artificial or forced.

Sutra 4 Even in the latter case, however, she should conduct herself as if her love were indeed natural, because men place their confidence in those women who apparently love them.

Sutra 5 In making her love known to the man, she should demonstrate she is free of avarice.

Sutra 6 And for the sake of her future credit she should refrain from acquiring money from him by unlawful means.

Sutra 7 A courtesan, well dressed and adorned with her ornaments, should sit or stand at the door of her house, and, without exposing herself too much, should be seen by the passers by, as if she were a commodity on view for sale.[1]

Sutra 8 She should form friendships with such persons as would enable her to draw men away from other women and attach them to her, to repair her own misfortunes, to acquire wealth, and to protect her from being bullied by those with whom she may have dealings.

Sutra 9 These persons are: officers of law and order; officials of the courts of justice; astrologers; powerful men, or men with interests; learned men; teachers of the sixty-four arts; *pithamarda*s or confidants; *vita*s or parasites; *vidushaka*s or jesters; flower sellers; perfumers; vendors of spirits; washermen; barbers; beggars; and such other persons as may be found necessary for the particular object to be acquired.

Sutra 10 The following kinds of men may be taken up with, simply for the purpose of getting their money:

Men of independent income
Young men
Men who are free from any ties
Men who hold positions of authority under the king
Men who have secured their means of livelihood without difficulty
Men possessed of unfailing sources of income
Men who consider themselves handsome
Men who are always boasting
Eunuchs who wish to be thought of as men
Men who have rivals
Men who are naturally generous
Men who have influence with the king or his ministers
Men who are always fortunate
Men who are proud of their wealth
Men who disobey the orders of their elders
Men upon whom the members of their caste keep an eye
Only sons whose fathers are wealthy

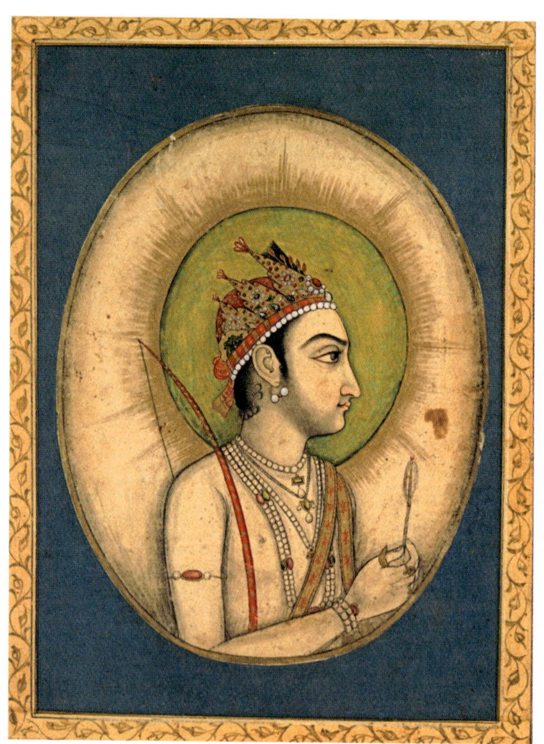

Ascetics who are internally troubled with desire
Brave men
Physicians of the king
Previous acquaintances

Sutra 11 On the other hand, those with excellent qualities are to be resorted to for the sake of love and fame. Such men are as follows:

Sutra 12 Men of high birth, learned, with a good knowledge of the world and doing the proper things at the proper times, poets, good storytellers, eloquent men, energetic men, men skilled in various arts, far-seeing into the future, possessed of great minds, full of perseverance, of a firm devotion, free from anger, liberal, affectionate to their parents, and with a liking for all social gatherings, skilled in completing verses begun by others and in various other sports, free from all disease, possessed of a perfect body, strong, and not addicted to drinking, powerful in sexual enjoyment, sociable, showing love toward women and attracting women's hearts to themselves, without being entirely devoted to them, possessed of an independent means of livelihood, free from envy, and, last of all, free from suspicion.

Such are the good qualities of a man.

Sutra 13 The woman should have the following characteristics:

Beauty and amiability, with auspicious marks on her body. She should have a liking for good qualities in other people, and also a liking for wealth. She should take delight in sexual unions resulting from love, and she should be of a firm mind and of the same class as the man with regard to sexual enjoyment.

She should always be anxious to acquire and obtain experience and knowledge, be free from avarice, and always have a liking for social gatherings and the arts.

Sutra 14 The following are the ordinary qualities of all women:

To be possessed of intelligence, good disposition and good manners; to be straightforward in behaviour and to be grateful; to have foresight; to be active, to be of consistent behaviour, and to have a knowledge of the proper times and places for doing things; always to speak without meanness, loud laughter, malignity, anger, avarice, dullness or stupidity; to have a knowledge of the *Kama Sutra*, and to be skilled in all the arts connected with it.

Sutra 15 The absence of any of the good qualities mentioned above is to be regarded as a fault in a woman.

Sutra 16 The following kinds of men are not fit to be resorted to by courtesans:

One who is consumptive; one who is sickly; one whose breath is foul; one whose wife is dear to him; one who speaks harshly; one who is always suspicious; one who is avaricious; one who is pitiless; one who is a thief; one who is self-conceited; one who has a liking for sorcery; one who does not care for respect or disrespect; one who can be won over, even by enemies, by money; and, lastly, one who is extremely bashful.

Sutra 17 Sages say that the motives of a courtesan are passion, fear, money, pleasure, returning some act of enmity, curiosity, sorrow, religious duty, fame, compassion, the desire to have a friend, shame, the likeness of the man to some beloved person, the search for good fortune, to get rid of the love of somebody else, the influence of birth and caste and neighbourhood, continued intimacy, and desire of dignity.

Sytra 18 But Vatsyayana asserts that the principal causes are material gain, escape from misfortune, and love.

Sutra 19 A courtesan should not sacrifice money to her love, because money is necessary for a courtesan's livelihood.

Sutra 20 But in cases of fear, and so on, she should pay regard to strength and other qualities.

Sutra 21 Moreover, even though she be invited by any man to join him, she should not at once consent to a union, because men are apt to despise things which are easily acquired.

Sutra 22 On such occasions she should first send the shampooers, and the singers and the jesters, who may be in her service, or, in their absence, the *pithamardas*, or confidants, and others, to find out the state of his feelings and the condition of his mind.

Sutra 23 By means of these persons she should ascertain whether the man is pure or impure, affected or the reverse, capable of attachment or indifferent, liberal or niggardly.

Sutra 24 And if she finds him to her liking, she should then employ the *vita* and others to attach his mind to her.

Sutra 25 Accordingly, the *pithamarda* should bring the man to her house under the pretence of seeing quail, cock or ram fights, hearing the myna talk, or seeing some other spectacle or art; or he may take the woman to the man's abode.

Sutra 26 After this, when the man comes to her house the woman should give him something capable of producing curiosity and love in his heart, such as an affectionate present, telling him that it was designed specially for his use.

Sutras 27–28 She should also amuse him for a long time by telling him stories and doing things that he may take the most delight in. When he goes away she should frequently send to him a female attendant skilled in carrying on a pleasant conversation with jokes, and also a small present at the same time. Whenever she can, she should accompany the *pithamarda* and go to his house herself under the pretence of some business or other.

Thus ends discussion of the means a courtesan can use to attach to herself the man desired.

Sutra 29 There are also some verses on the subject as follows:
"When a lover comes to her abode, a courtesan should give him a mixture of betel leaves and betel nut, garlands of flowers and perfumed ointments, and should entertain him with a conversation."

Sutra 30 "She should also give him some loving presents, and make an exchange of her own things with his, and at the same time should show him her skill in sexual enjoyment."

Sutra 31 "When a courtesan is thus united with her lover she should always delight him by affectionate gifts, conversation and the application of tender means of enjoyment."

Chapter II Living like a wife

Sutras 1–2 When a courtesan is living as a wife with her lover, she should behave like a chaste woman and do everything to his satisfaction. Her duty in this respect is, in short, that she should give him pleasure but should not become attached to him, though behaving as if she were really attached.

Sutra 3 The following is the manner in which she is to conduct herself, so as to accomplish the aforementioned purpose. She should have a mother dependent on her, one who should appear to be harsh and who looks upon money as her chief object in life. In the event of there being no mother, then an old and confidential nurse should play the same role.

Sutras 4–5 The mother or nurse, for their part, should appear to be displeased with the lover and forcibly take her away from him. The woman herself should always show pretended anger, dejection, fear and shame on this account, but should not disobey the mother or nurse at any time.

Sutras 6–7 She should make out to the mother or nurse that the man is suffering from bad health, and making this a pretext for going to see him, she should go on that account.

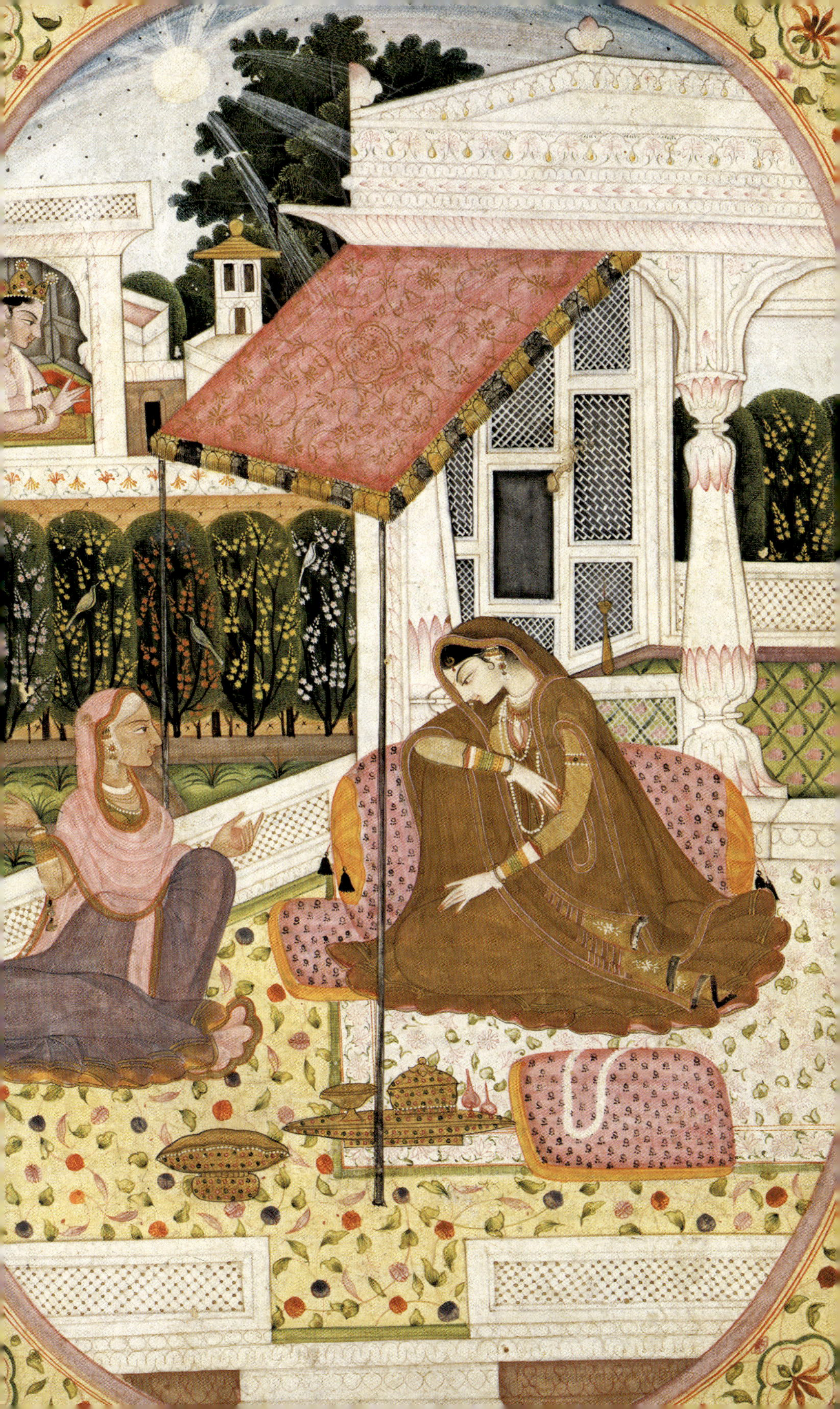

She is, moreover, to do the following things for the purpose of gaining the man's favour:

Sutra 8 Send her female attendant to bring the flowers used by him on the previous day in order that she may use them as a mark of affection, also to ask for the betel leaf mixture uneaten by him.

Sutra 9 Express wonder at his knowledge of sexual intercourse; show readiness to learn from him the sixty-four kinds of pleasure mentioned by Babhravya; continually practise the ways of enjoyment as taught by him, and according to his liking; keep his secrets; tell him her own desires and secrets; conceal her anger; never neglect him on the bed when he turns his face toward her; touch any parts of his body according to his wish; and kiss and embrace him when he is asleep.

Sutra 10 Look at him with apparent anxiety when he is rapt in thought, or thinking of some subject other than her; show neither complete shamelessness nor excessive bashfulness when he meets her, or sees her standing on the terrace of her house from the public road; hate his enemies; love those who are dear to him; show a liking for that which he likes; be in high or low spirits according to the state that he is in; express a curiosity to see his wives; not continue her anger for a long time; and if she is concerned he has another attachment, she should tell him she suspects even the marks and wounds made by herself with her nails and teeth on his body to have been made by some other woman.

Sutras 11–12 Keep her love for him unexpressed by words, but show it by deeds, signs and hints; remain silent when he is asleep, intoxicated or sick; be attentive when he describes his good actions, and recite them afterwards to his praise and benefit; give witty replies to him if he be sufficiently attached to her.

Sutra 13 Listen to all his stories, except those that relate to her rivals.

Sutra 14 Express feelings of dejection and sorrow if he sighs, yawns or falls down.

Sutra 15 Pronounce the words "live long" when he sneezes.

Sutra 16 Pretend to be ill, or to have the desire of pregnancy, when she feels dejected.

Sutra 17 Refrain from praising the good qualities of anybody else, and from censuring those who possess the same faults as her own man; wear anything that may have been given to her by him.

Sutra 18 Refrain from putting on ornaments, and from taking food, when he is in pain, sick, low-spirited or suffering from misfortune.

Sutra 19 And condole and lament with him over the same; wish to accompany him if he happens to leave the country or if he be banished from it by the king; express a desire not to live after him.

Sutra 20 Tell him that the whole object and desire of her life was to be united with him; offer previously promised sacrifices to the gods when he acquires wealth, or has some desire fulfilled, or when he has recovered from some illness or disease.

Sutra 21 Put on ornaments every day; not act too freely with him.

Sutra 22–23 Recite his name and the name of his family in her songs; place his hand on her loins, bosom and forehead, and fall asleep after feeling the pleasure of his touch; sit on his lap and fall asleep there.

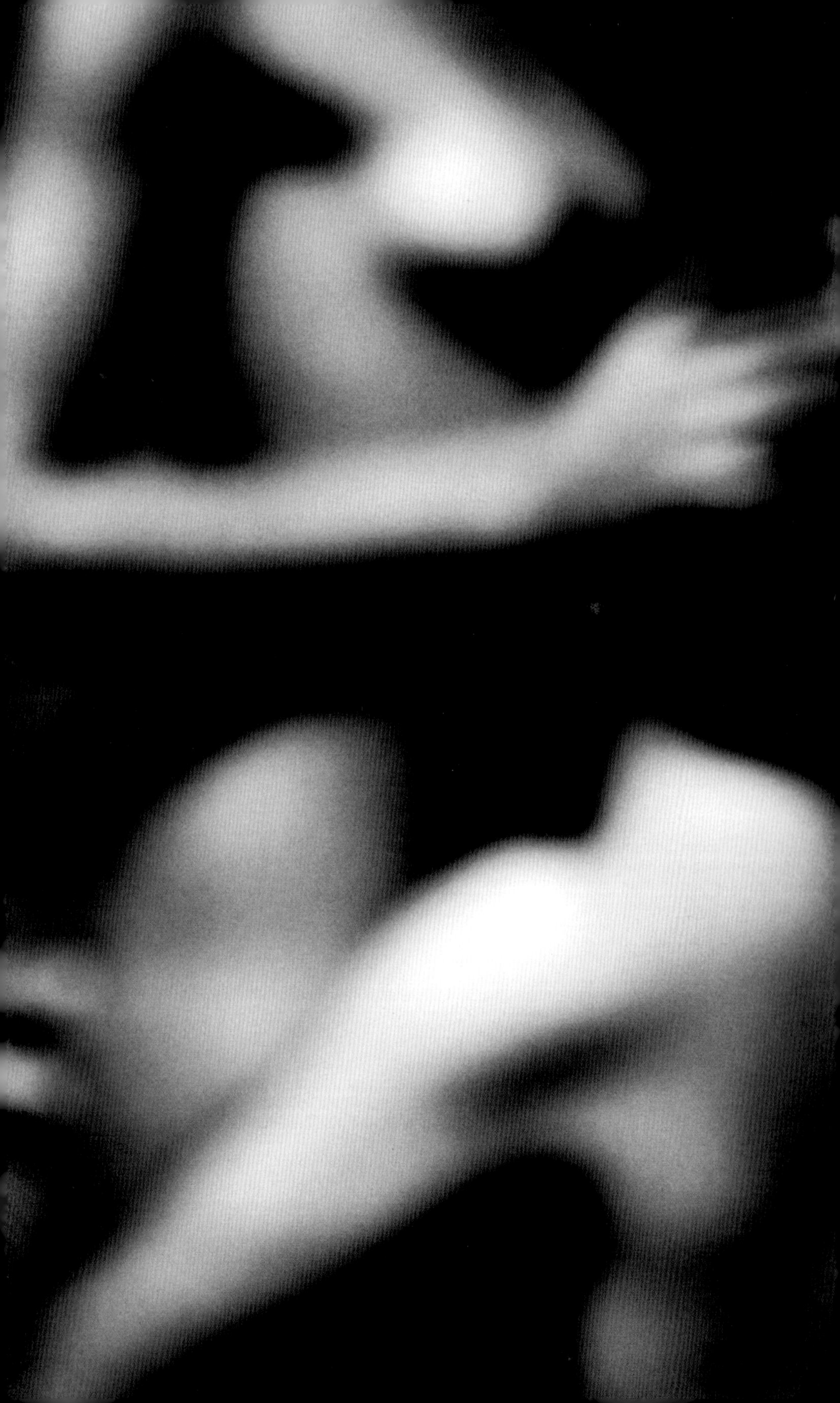

Sutra 24 Wish to have a child by him; desire not to live longer than him.

Sutra 25 Refrain from revealing his secrets to others.

Sutra 26–27 Dissuade him from vows and fasts by saying "let the sin fall upon me"; keep vows and fasts along with him when it is impossible to change his mind on the subject; tell him that vows and fasts are difficult to be observed, even by herself, when she has any dispute with him about them.

Sutras 28–30 Look on her own wealth and his without any distinction; abstain from going to public assemblies without him, and accompany him when he desires her to do so; take delight in using things previously used by him, and in eating food that he has left uneaten.

Sutra 31 Venerate his family, his disposition, his skill in the arts, his learning, his caste, his complexion, his native country, his friends, his good qualities, his age and his sweet temper.

Sutra 32 Ask him to sing, and to do other such things, if able to.

Sutra 33 Go to him without paying any regard to fear, to cold, to heat or to rain.

Sutra 34 Say with regard to the next world that he should be her lover even there.

Sutras 35–36 Adapt her tastes, disposition and actions to his liking; abstain from sorcery.

Sutras 37–38 Dispute continually with her mother on the subject of going to him, and, when forcibly taken by her mother to some other place, express her desire to die by taking poison, by starving herself to death, by stabbing herself with some weapon, or by hanging herself.

Sutra 39 And lastly assure the man of her constancy and love by means of her agents.

Sutras 40–42 Receive money herself, but refrain from any dispute with her mother with regard to pecuniary matters.

Sutra 43 When the man sets out on a journey, she should make him swear that he will return quickly.

Sutra 44 In his absence she should put aside her vows of worship and should wear no ornaments except those that are lucky.

Sutra 45 If the time for his return has passed, she should endeavour to ascertain the real time of his return from omens, from the reports of people, and from the positions of the planets, the moon and the stars.

Sutra 46 On occasions of amusement, and of auspicious dreams, she should say, "Let me be soon reunited with him".

Sutra 47 If, moreover, she feels melancholy, or sees any inauspicious omen, she should perform some rite to appease the god of love.

Sutras 48–50 When the man does return home she should worship the god of love and offer oblations to other deities, and have a pot filled with water brought to her in the company of her friends.

Sutra 51 She should feed crows as a token of her oblations.

Sutras 52–53 After the first visit is over she should ask her lover also to perform certain rites, which he will do if he is sufficiently attached to her.

Sutra 54 Now a man is said to be sufficiently attached to a woman when his love is disinterested; when he has the same object in view as his beloved one; when he is quite free from any suspicions on her account; and when he is indifferent to money with regard to her.

Sutra 55 Such is the manner of a courtesan living with a man like a wife, and set forth here from the rules of Dattaka for the sake of guidance. What is not laid down here should be practised according to the custom of the people and the nature of each individual man.

Sutra 56 There are also two verses on the subject as follows:

"The extent of the love of women is not known, even to those who are the objects of their affection, on account of its subtlety, and on account of the avarice and natural intelligence of womankind."

Sutra 57 "Women are hardly ever known in their true light, though they may love men, or become indifferent toward them, may give them delight, or abandon them, or may extract from them all the wealth that they may possess."

Chapter III The means of getting money; the signs of the change of a lover's feelings; and the way to get rid of him

Sutra 1 Money is extracted from a lover in two ways: by natural or lawful means, and by artifices.

Sutra 2 The learned sages were of the opinion that when a courtesan can get as much money as she wants from her lover, she should not make use of artifice.

Sutra 3 But according to Vatsyayana, although she may get some money from him by natural means, when she makes use of artifice he gives her double, and therefore artifice should be resorted to for the purpose of extorting money from him in any event.

The artifices to be used for getting money from her lover are as follows:

Sutra 4 When taking money from him on different occasions – for the purpose of purchasing ornaments, food, drink, flowers, perfumes and clothes – either do not buy them, or get from him more than their cost.

Sutra 5 Praising his intelligence to his face.

Sutra 6 Pretending to be obliged to make gifts on occasion of festivals connected with vows, trees, gardens, temples or tanks.[2]

Sutra 7 Pretending that at the time of going to his house, her jewels have been stolen either by the king's guards or by robbers.

Sutra 8 Alleging that her property has been destroyed by fire, by the house collapsing, or by the carelessness of her servants.

Sutra 9 Pretending to have lost the ornaments of her lover along with her own.

Sutra 10 Causing him to hear through other people of the expenses incurred by her in coming to see him.

Sutra 11 Contracting debts for the sake of her lover, and disputing with

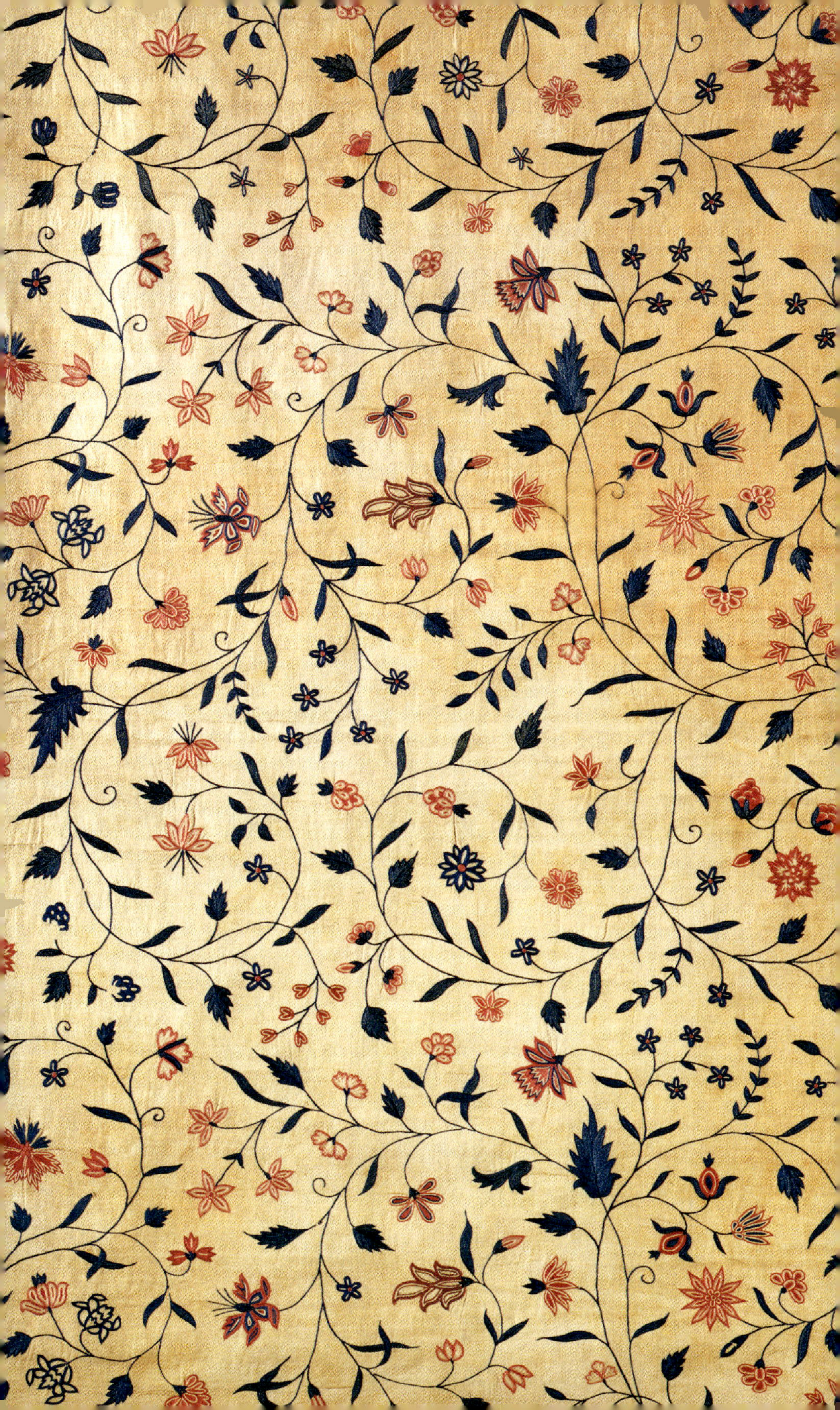

her mother on account of some expense incurred by her for her lover, and which was not approved of by her mother.

Sutra 12 Not going to parties and festivities in the houses of her friends for the want of presents to make to them, having previously informed her lover of the valuable presents given to her by these friends.

Sutra 13 Not performing certain festive rites under the pretence that she has no money to perform them with.

Sutra 14 Engaging artists to do something for her lover.

Sutra 15 Entertaining physicians and ministers for the purpose of attaining some object.

Sutra 16 Assisting friends and benefactors in time of misfortune.

Sutra 17 Performing household rites.

Having to pay the wedding expenses of the son of a female friend.

Having to satisfy curious wishes including her state of pregnancy.

Pretending to be ill, and charging the cost of treatment.

Having to alleviate a friend's troubles.

Sutra 18 Selling some of her ornaments to give her lover a present.

Sutra 19 Pretending to sell some of her ornaments, furniture or cooking utensils to a trader, who has been tutored how to behave.

Sutra 20 Having to buy cooking utensils of greater value than those of other people, so that they might be more easily distinguished and not changed for others of an inferior description.

Sutra 21 Remembering the former favours of her lover, and causing them always to be spoken of by her friends and followers.

Sutra 22 Informing her lover of the great gains of other courtesans.

Sutra 23 Describing before them, and in the presence of her lover, her own great gains, and making them out to be greater even than theirs, though such may not have been really the case.

Sutra 24 Openly opposing her mother when her mother endeavours to persuade her to take up with men with whom she has been formerly acquainted, on account of the great gains to be got from them.

Sutras 25–26 Pointing out to her lover the liberality of his rivals.

Thus ends consideration of the ways and means of a courtesan getting money.

Sutra 27 A woman should always know the state of mind, the feelings and the disposition of her lover toward her from the changes of his temper, his manner and the colour of his face.

The behaviour of a lover who is becoming indifferent is as follows:

Sutra 28 He gives the woman either less than is wanted, or something else than that which is asked for.

Sutra 29 He keeps her in hopes by promises.

Sutra 30 He pretends to do one thing, and does something else.

Sutra 31 He does not fulfil her desires.

Sutra 32 He forgets to honour his promises, or does something else than that which he has promised.

Sutra 33 He speaks with his own servants in a mysterious and unintelligible way.

Sutra 34 He sleeps elsewhere – at the house of another courtesan – under the pretence of having to do something for a friend.

Sutra 35 He speaks in private with the attendants of a woman with whom he was formerly acquainted.

Sutras 36–38 Now, when a courtesan finds that her lover's disposition toward her is changing, she should get possession of all his best things before he becomes aware of her intentions, and allow a supposed creditor to take them away forcibly from her in satisfaction of some pretended debt.

Sutra 39 After this, if the lover is rich and has always behaved well toward her, she should treat him with respect.

Sutra 40 But if he is poor and destitute, she should get rid of him as if she had never been acquainted with him in any way before.

The means of getting rid of a lover are as follows:

Sutra 41 Describing the habits and vices of the lover as disagreeable and censurable, with the sneer of the lip and the stamp of the foot.

Speaking on a subject with which he is not acquainted.

Showing no admiration for his learning, and passing adverse remarks.

Putting down his pride.

Seeking the company of men who are superior to him in wisdom.

Showing a disregard for him on all occasions.

Censuring men possessed of the same faults as her lover.

Expressing dissatisfaction at the ways and means of enjoyment used by him.

Sutra 42 Not giving him her mouth to kiss.

Refusing access to her *jaghana*; that is, the part of the body between the navel and the thighs.

Showing a dislike for the wounds made by his nails and teeth.

Not pressing close up against him at the time when he embraces her.

Keeping her limbs still at the time of congress.

Desiring him to enjoy her when he is fatigued.

Laughing at his attachment to her.

Not responding to his embraces.

Turning away from him when be begins to embrace her.

Pretending to be sleepy.

Going out visiting, or into company, when she perceives his desire to enjoy her during the daytime.

Sutra 43 Misconstruing his words.

Laughing without any joke, or, at the time of any joke made by him, laughing under some pretence.

Looking with glances at her own attendants, and clapping her hands when he says anything.

Interrupting him in the middle of his stories, and beginning to tell other stories herself.

Reciting his faults and his vices, and declaring them to be incurable.

Saying words to her female attendants calculated to cut the heart of her lover to the quick.

Sutra 44 Taking care not to look at him when he comes to her.

Asking him what cannot be granted.
And, after all, finally dismissing him.

Sutra 45 There are also two verses on this subject as follows:
"The duty of a courtesan consists in forming connections with suitable men after due and full consideration, and attaching the person with whom she is united to herself; in obtaining wealth from the person who is attached to her, and then dismissing him after she has taken away all his possessions."

Sutra 46 "A courtesan leading in this manner the life of a wife is not troubled with too many lovers, and yet obtains abundance of wealth."

Chapter IV About reunion with a former lover

Sutra 1 When a courtesan abandons her present lover after all his wealth is exhausted, she may then consider reunion with a former lover.

Sutra 2 But she should return to him only if he has acquired fresh wealth, or is still wealthy, and if he is still attached to her.

Sutra 3 And if this man be living at the time with some other woman she should ponder the matter and reach a considered decision before she acts.

Now such a man has to belong to one of the six following categories:

Sutra 4 He may have left the first woman of his own accord, and may even have left another woman since then.

Sutra 5 He may have been driven away from both women.

Sutra 6 He may have left the one woman of her own accord, and been driven away by the other.

Sutra 7 He may have left the one woman of his own accord, and be living with another woman.

Sutra 8 He may have been driven away from the one woman, and left the other of his own accord.

Sutra 9 He may have been driven away by the one woman, and may be living with another.

Sutra 10 Now if the man has left both women of his own accord, he should not be resorted to, on account of the fickleness of his mind and his indifference to the excellences of both of them.

Sutra 11 As regards the man who may have been driven away from both women, if he has been driven away from the last one because the woman could get more money from some other man, then he should be resorted to, for if attached to the first woman he would give her more money through vanity and emulation to spite the other woman.

Sutra 12 But if he has been driven away by the woman on account of his poverty, or stinginess, he should not then be resorted to.

Sutra 13 In the case of the man who may have left the one woman of his own accord, and been driven away by the other, if he agrees to return to the former and give her plenty of money beforehand, then he should be resorted to.

Sutra 14 In the case of the man who may have left the one woman of his own accord, and be living with another woman, the former (wishing to take up with him again) should first ascertain if he left her in the first instance in the hope of finding some particular excellence in the other woman, and that not having found any such excellence, he was willing to come back to her, and to give her much money on account of his conduct, and on account of his affection still existing for her.

Sutra 15 Or, whether, having discovered many faults in the other woman, he would now see even more excellences in herself than actually exist, and would be prepared to give her much money for these qualities.

Sutra 16 Or, lastly, to consider whether he was a weak man, or a man fond of enjoying many women, or one who liked a poor woman, or one who never did anything for the woman that he was with. After maturely considering all these things, she should resort to him or not, according to circumstances.

Sutras 17–20 As regards the man who may have been driven away from the one woman, and left the other of his own accord, the former woman (wishing to reunite with him) should first ascertain whether he still has any affection for her, and would consequently spend much money upon her; or whether, being attached to her excellent qualities, he did not take delight in any other woman; or whether, being driven away from her formerly before completely satisfying his sexual desires, he wished to get back to her, so as to be revenged for the injury done to him; or whether he wished to create confidence in her mind, and then take back from her the wealth which she formerly took from him, and finally destroy her; or, lastly, whether he wished first to separate her from her present lover, and then to break away from her himself.
If, after considering all these things, she is of the opinion that his intentions are really pure and honest, she can reunite herself with him.

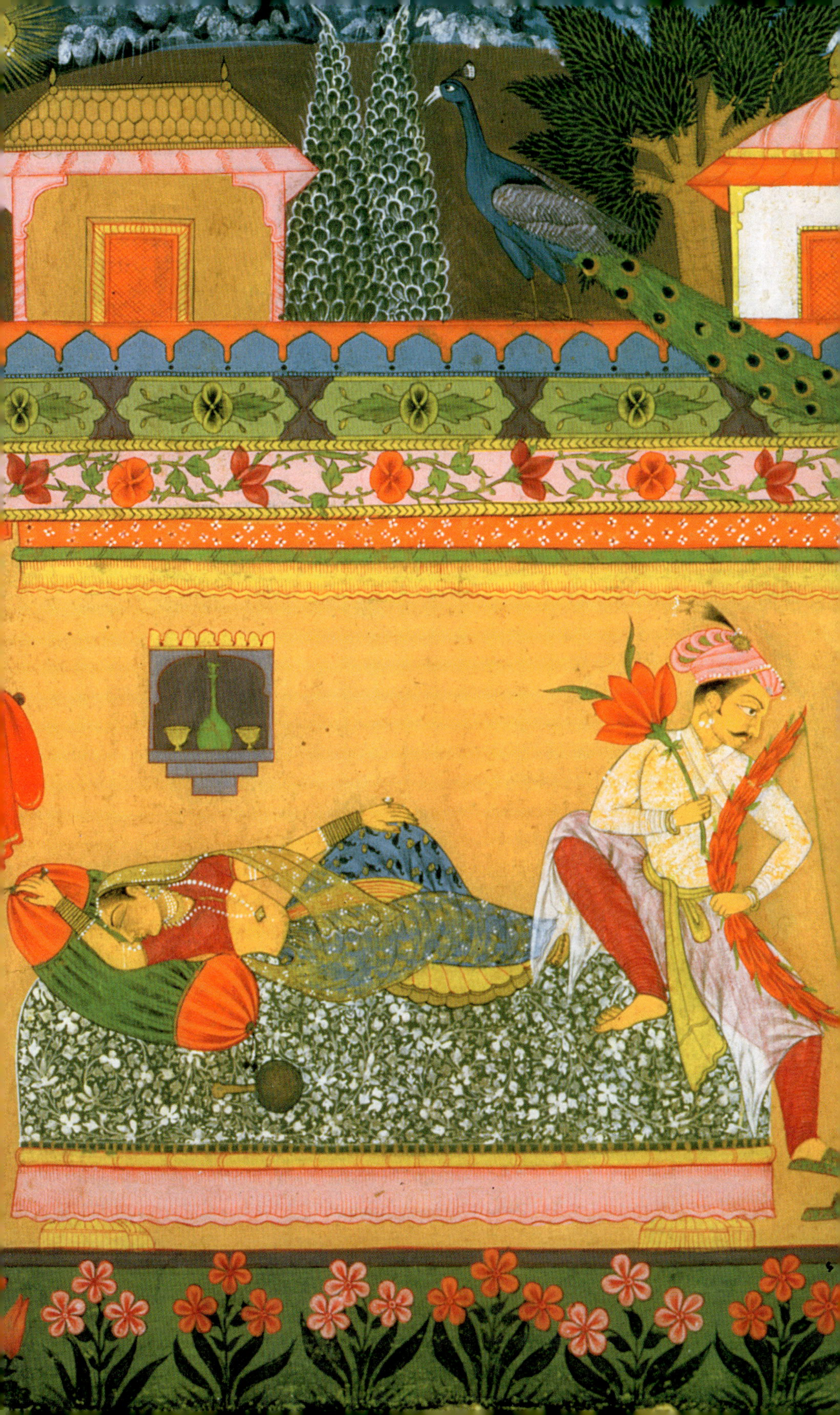

But if his mind be at all tainted with evil intentions, he should be avoided.

Sutras 21–23 In the case of the man who may have been driven away by one woman, and be living with another, if the man makes overtures to return to the first one, the courtesan should consider well before she acts, and while the other woman is engaged in attracting him to herself, she should try in her turn (though keeping herself behind the scenes) to win him over, on the grounds of any of the following considerations:

Sutra 24 That he was driven away unjustly and for no proper reason, and now that he has gone to another woman every effort must be used to bring him back to myself.

Sutra 25 That if he were once to converse with me again, he would break away from the other woman.

Sutra 26 That the pride of my present lover would be put down by means of the former one.

Sutra 27 That he has become wealthy, has secured a higher position and holds a place of authority under the king.

That he is separate from his wife.

That he is now independent.

That he lives apart from his father or brother.

Sutra 28 That by making peace with him, I shall be able to secure a very rich man, who is prevented from coming to me by my present lover.

Sutra 29 That because he is not respected by his wife, I shall now be able to separate him from her.

Sutra 30 That the friend of this man loves my rival, who hates me cordially; I shall therefore by this means separate the friend from his mistress.

Sutra 31 And lastly, I shall bring discredit upon him by bringing him back to me, thus showing the fickleness of his mind.

Sutra 32 When a courtesan is resolved to take up again with a former lover, her *pithamarda* and other servants should tell him that his former expulsion from the woman's house was caused by the wickedness of her mother; that the woman loved him just as much as ever at that time, but could not help the occurrence on account of her deference to her mother's will.

Sutra 33 That she hated the union of her present lover, and disliked him excessively.

Sutra 34 In addition to this, they should create confidence in his mind by speaking to him of her former love for him, and should allude to the mark of that love that she has always remembered.

Sutra 35 This mark of her love should be connected with some kind of pleasure that may have been practised by him, such as his way of kissing her, or his manner of having a connection with her.

Thus ends discussion of the ways of bringing about a reunion with a former lover.

Sutra 36 When a woman has to choose between two lovers, one of whom was formerly united with her, while the other is a stranger, the *acharya*s (sages) are of the opinion that the first is preferable: because his disposition and character are already known, he can be easily satisfied.

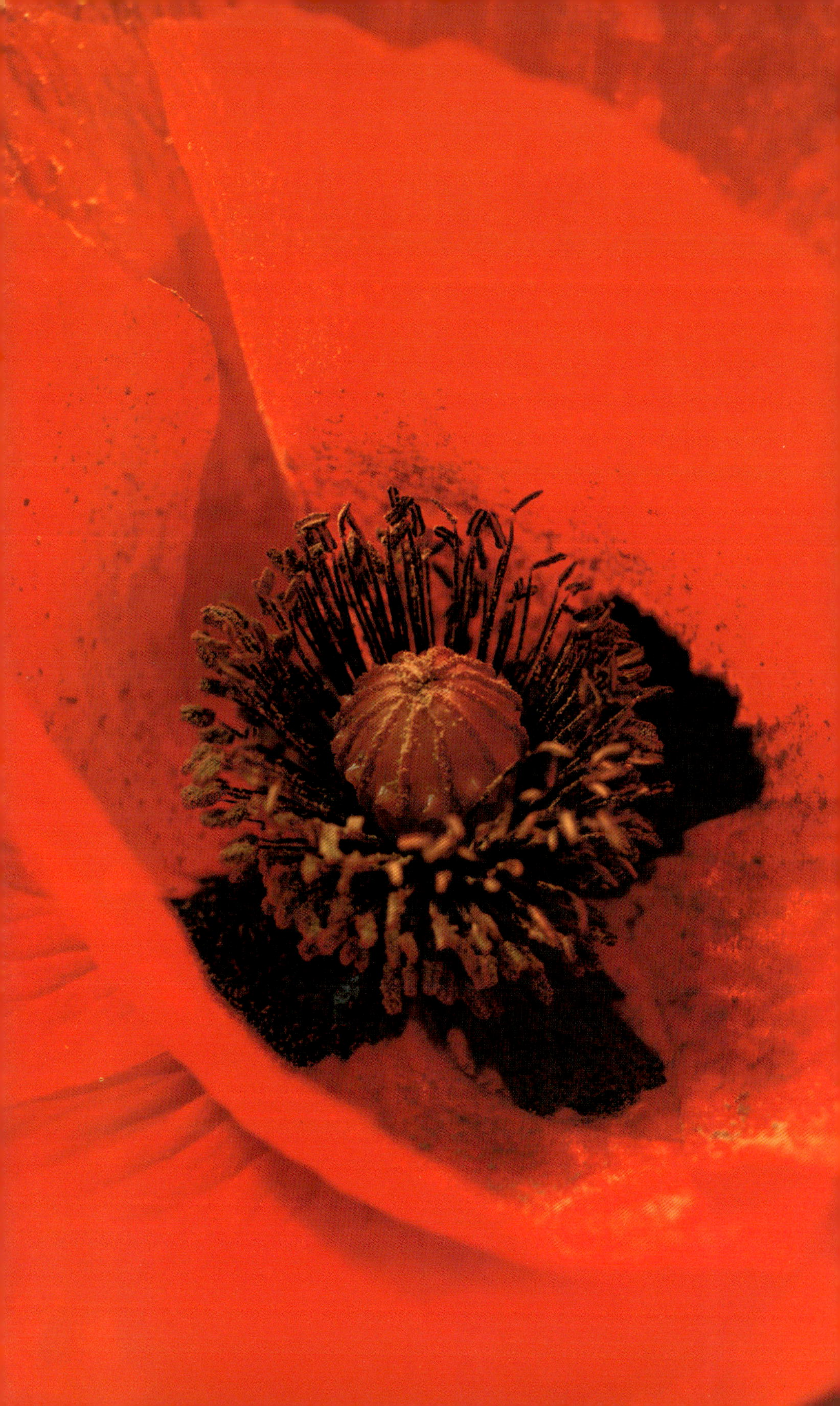

Sutra 37 But Vatsyayana thinks that a former lover, having already spent a great deal of his wealth, is not able or willing to give much money again, and is not therefore to be relied upon so much as a stranger.

Sutra 38 Particular cases may however arise differing from this general rule on account of the different natures of men.

Sutra 39 There are also verses on the subject as follows: "Reunion with a former lover may be desirable so as to separate some particular woman from some particular man, or some particular man from some particular woman, or to have a certain effect upon the present lover."

Sutra 40 "When a man is excessively attached to a woman, he is afraid of her coming into contact with other men; he does not then regard or notice her faults and he gives her much wealth through fear of her leaving him."

Sutra 41 "A courtesan should be agreeable to the man who is attached to her, and despise the man who does not care for her."

Sutra 42 "If while she is living with one man, a messenger comes to her from some other man, she may either refuse to listen to any negotiations on his part, or appoint a fixed time for him to visit her."

Sutra 43 "But she should not leave the man who may be living with her and who may be attached to her."

Sutra 44 "A wise woman should only renew her connection with a former lover if she is satisfied that good fortune, gain, love and friendship are likely to be the result of such a reunion."

Chapter V Different kinds of gain

Sutra 1 When a courtesan is able to realize much money every day, by having many customers, she should not confine herself to a single lover.

Sutras 2–4 Under such circumstances, she should fix her rate for one night, after considering the place, the season and the condition of the people, and having regard to her own good qualities and good looks, and after comparing her rates with those of other courtesans. She can inform her lovers, friends and acquaintances about these charges. If, however, she can obtain a great gain from a single lover, she may resort to him alone, and live with him like a wife.

Sutra 5 The sages believe that when a courtesan has the chance of an equal gain from two lovers at the same time, a preference should be given to the one who would give her the kind of thing she wants.

Sutra 6 But Vatsyayana says that the preference should be given to the one who gives her gold, because it cannot be taken back like some other things, it can be easily received, and it is also the means of procuring anything that may be wished for.

Sutra 7 Of such things as gold, silver, copper, bronze, iron, pots, furniture, beds, blankets, silk, fragrant substances, ghee, oil, corn, cattle, and other things of a like nature, the first is superior to all the others.

Sutra 8 When the same labour is required to gain any two lovers, or when the same kind of thing is to be got from each of them, the choice should be made by the advice of a friend, or it may be made from their personal qualities, or from the signs of good or bad fortune that may be connected with them.

Sutra 9 When there are two lovers, one of whom is attached to the courtesan, and the other is simply very generous, the sages say that preference should be given to the generous lover.

Sutra 10 But Vatsyayana is of the opinion that the one who is really attached to the courtesan should be preferred, because he can be made to be generous. If the person is a miser he can be induced to part with money and gifts if he becomes fond of a woman, but a man who is simply generous cannot be made to love with real attachment. But among those who are attached to her, if there is one who is poor and one who is rich, the preference is to be given to the latter.

Sutra 11 When there are two lovers, one of whom is generous, and the other ready to do any service for the courtesan, some sages say that the one who is ready to do any service should be preferred.

Sutra 12 But Vatsyayana is of the opinion that a man who does a service thinks that his object will be indebted to him when he has done something once, but a generous man does not care for what he has given before.

Sutra 13 Even here the choice should be guided by the likelihood of the future good to be derived from her union with either of them.

Sutra 14 When one of the two lovers is grateful, and the other liberal, some sages say that the liberal one should be preferred.

Sutra 15 But Vatsyayana is of the opinion that the former should be chosen, because liberal men are generally haughty, plain spoken and wanting in consideration towards others. Even though these liberal men have been on friendly terms for a long time, if they see any fault in the courtesan, or are told lies about her by some other woman, they do not care for past services, but leave abruptly. On the other hand the grateful man does not break off from her at once, on account of a regard for the pains she may have taken to please him.

Sutra 16 In this case also the choice is to be guided with respect to what may happen in future.

Sutra 17 When an occasion for complying with the request of a friend and a chance of getting money come together, the sages say that the chance of getting money should be preferred.

Sutras 18–19 But Vatsyayana thinks that the money can be obtained tomorrow as well as today, but if the request of a friend be not at once complied with, he may become disaffected. Even here, in making the choice, regard must be paid to future good fortune.

Sutra 20 On such an occasion, however, the courtesan might pacify her friend by pretending to have some work to do, and telling him that his request will be complied with next day, and in this way secure the chance of getting the money that has been offered her.

Sutra 21 When the chance of getting money and the chance of avoiding some disaster come at the same time, the sages are of the opinion that the chance of getting money should be preferred.

Sutra 22 But Vatsyayana says that money has only a limited importance, while a disaster that is once averted may never occur again.

Sutras 23–24 Here, however, the choice should be guided by the greatness or smallness of the disaster.

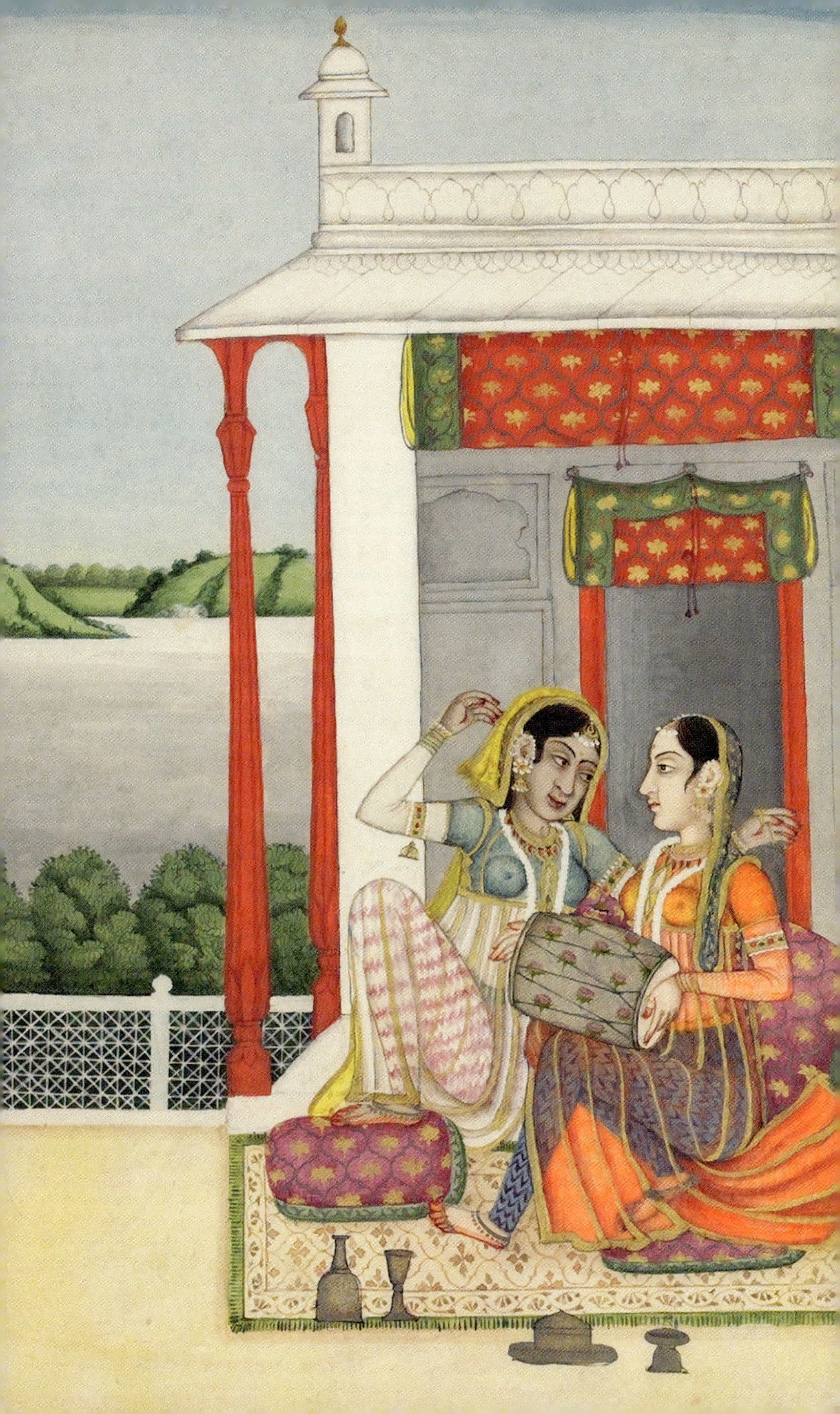

The money gained by the wealthiest and best kind of courtesans should be spent as follows:

Sutra 25 Constructing temples, tanks, gardens, groves and bridges; giving 1,000 cows to different Brahmins; providing for the worship of the gods, collecting donations and celebrating festivals in their honour; and, lastly, performing such vows as may be within their means.

The money gained by other courtesans whose livelihood depends on physical charms should be spent as follows:

Sutras 26–27 Having a white dress to wear every day; getting sufficient food and drink to satisfy hunger and thirst; eating a perfumed *tambula*[3] daily; and wearing gilded ornaments.

Sutra 28 The sages say that these represent the gains of all the middle and lower classes of courtesans.

Sutra 29 But Vatsyayana is of the opinion that their gains cannot be calculated, or fixed in any way, as these depend on the influence of the place, the customs of the people, their appearance, and other things.

Sutras 30–31 When a courtesan wants to keep some particular man from another woman; or wishes to get him away from a woman to whom he may be attached, or to deprive a woman of the gains realized by her from him; or if she thinks that she would raise her position or enjoy some great good fortune or become desirable to all men by uniting herself with this man; or if she wishes to get his assistance in averting some misfortune; or is really attached to him and loves him; or wishes to injure somebody through his means; or has regard to some former favour conferred upon her by him; or wishes to be united with him merely from desire; for any of the above reasons, she should agree to take from him only a small sum of money in a friendly way.

Sutra 32 When a courtesan intends to abandon a particular lover, and take up with another one, or when she has reason to believe that her lover will shortly leave her and return to his wives, or that, having squandered all his money and become penniless, he is about to be taken away by his guardian, or master, or father, or that he is about to lose his position soon, or, lastly, that he is of a very fickle mind, she should, under any of these circumstances, endeavour to get as much money as she can from him as soon as possible.

Sutra 33 On the other hand, when the courtesan thinks that her lover is about to receive valuable presents, or get a place of authority from the king, or be close to inheriting a fortune, or that his ship will soon arrive laden with merchandise, or that he has large stocks of corn and other commodities, or that if anything was done for him it would not be done in vain, or that he is always true to his word, then she should have regard to her future welfare and live with the man like a wife.

Sutra 34 There are also verses on the subject as follows: "In considering her present gains, and her future welfare, a courtesan should avoid such persons as have won their means of subsistence with very great difficulty, as also those who have become selfish and hard-hearted by becoming the favourites of kings."

Sutra 35 "She should make every endeavour to unite herself with prosperous and well-to-do people, and with those whom it is dangerous to avoid, or to slight in any way. Even at some cost to herself she should become acquainted with energetic and liberal-minded men, who when pleased would give her a large sum of money, even for very little service, or for some small thing."

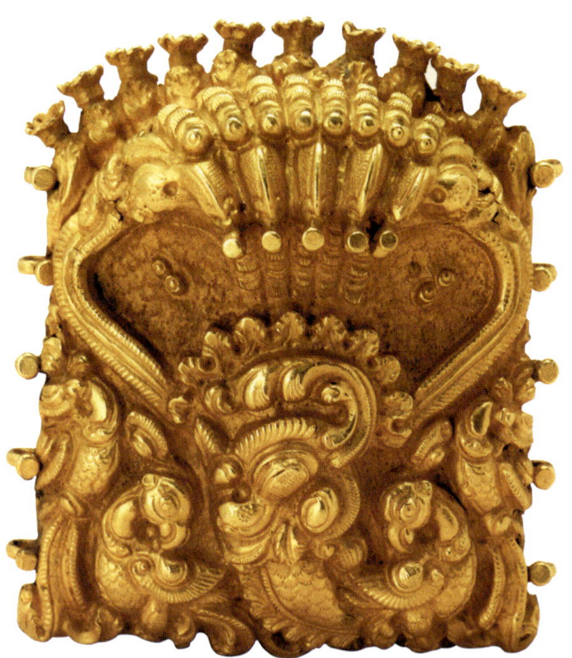

Chapter VI Gains and losses; attendant gains and losses; doubts; and the different kinds of courtesans

Sutra 1 It sometimes happens that while gains are being sought for, or expected to be realized, losses are the result of our efforts.

Sutra 2 The causes of these losses are:

Weakness of intellect
Excessive love
Excessive pride
Excessive self-conceit
Excessive simplicity
Excessive confidence
Excessive anger
Carelessness
Recklessness
Influence of an evil genius

Sutra 3 The results of these losses are:

Expense incurred without any result
Destruction of future good fortune
Stoppage of gains about to be realized
Loss of what has already been obtained
Acquisition of a sour temper
Becoming unamiable to everybody
Injury to health
Loss of hair and other accidents

Sutra 4 The courtesan should therefore shun the company of people who influence her adversely in this way.

Sutra 5 Now gain is of three kinds: gain of wealth, gain of religious merit, and gain of pleasure. And similarly loss is of three kinds: loss of wealth, loss of religious merit, and loss of pleasure.

Sutra 6 At the time when gains are sought, if other gains come along with them, these are called "attendant gains".

Sutra 7 When gain is uncertain, the doubt of its being a gain is called a "simple doubt".

Sutra 8 When there is a doubt whether either of two things will happen or not, it is called a "mixed doubt".

Sutra 9 If while one thing is being done two results take place, it is called a "combination of two results".

Sutra 10 And if several results follow from the same action, it is called a "combination of results on every side". We shall now give examples.

Sutras 11–12 As already stated, gain and loss are each of three kinds.

When by living with a great man a courtesan acquires present wealth, and in addition to this becomes acquainted with other people, and thus obtains a chance of future fortune, and becomes desirable to all, this is called a "gain of wealth attended by other gain".

Sutra 13 When by living with a man a courtesan simply gets money, this is called a "gain of wealth not attended by any other gain".

Sutra 14 When a courtesan receives money from other people besides her lover, the results are: the chance of the loss of future good from her present lover; the chance of disaffection of a man securely attached to her; the hatred of all; and the chance of a union with some low person, tending to destroy her future good. This gain is called a "gain of wealth attended by losses".

Sutra 15 When a courtesan, at her own expense and without any results in the shape of gain, has connection with a great man, or an avaricious minister, for the sake of diverting some misfortune, or removing some cause that may be threatening the destruction of a great gain, this loss is said to be a "loss of wealth attended by gains of the future good which it may bring about".

Sutra 16 When a courtesan is kind, even at her own expense, to a man who is very stingy, or to a man proud of his looks, or to an ungrateful man skilled in gaining the hearts of others, without any good resulting from these connections to her in the end, this loss is called a "loss of wealth not attended by any gain".

Sutra 17 When a courtesan is kind to any such man as described above, but who in addition is a favourite of the king, and moreover cruel and powerful, without any good result in the end, and with a chance of her being turned away at any moment, this loss is called a "loss of wealth attended by other losses".

Sutras 18–19 In this way gains and losses, and attendant gains and losses in religious merit and pleasures, may become known to the reader, and combinations of all of them may also be made.

Thus end the remarks on gains and losses and attendant gains and losses.

Sutra 20 In the next place we come to doubts, which are again of three kinds: doubts about wealth, doubts about religious merit, and doubts about pleasures. The following are examples:

When a courtesan is not certain how much a man may give her, or spend upon her, this is called a "doubt about wealth".

Sutra 21 When a courtesan feels doubtful whether she is right in entirely abandoning a lover from whom she is unable to get money, having taken all his wealth from him in the first instance, this doubt is called a "doubt about religious merit".

Sutra 22 When a courtesan is unable to get hold of a lover to her liking, and is uncertain whether she will derive any pleasure from a person surrounded by his family, or from a low person, this is called a "doubt about pleasure".

Sutra 23 When a courtesan is uncertain whether some powerful but low-principled fellow would cause loss to her on account of her not being civil to him this is called a "doubt about the loss of wealth".

Sutra 24 When a courtesan feels doubtful whether she would lose religious merit by abandoning a man who is attached to her without giving him the slightest favour, and thereby causing him unhappiness in this world and the next,[4] this doubt is called a "doubt about the loss of religious merit".

Sutra 25 When a courtesan is uncertain as to whether she might create disaffection by speaking out to reveal her love and thus not get her desire satisfied, this is called a "doubt about the loss of pleasure".

Thus end the remarks on simple doubts.

Sutra 26 Now follows a description of mixed doubts:

Sutra 27 The intercourse or connection with a stranger whose disposition is unknown, and who may have been introduced by a lover, or by one who possesses authority, may produce either gain or loss, and therefore this is called a "mixed doubt about the gain or loss of wealth".

Sutra 28 When a courtesan is requested by a friend, or is impelled by pity to have intercourse with a learned Brahmin, a religious student, a sacrificer, a devotee or an ascetic who may have fallen in love with her, and who may be consequently at the point of death, by doing this she might either gain or lose religious merit, and therefore this is called a "mixed doubt about the gain or loss of religious merit".

Sutra 29 If a courtesan relies solely upon the report of other people (that is, hearsay) about a man, and goes to him without ascertaining herself whether he possesses good qualities or not, she may either gain or lose pleasure in proportion as he may be good or bad, and therefore this is called a "mixed doubt about the gain or loss of pleasure".

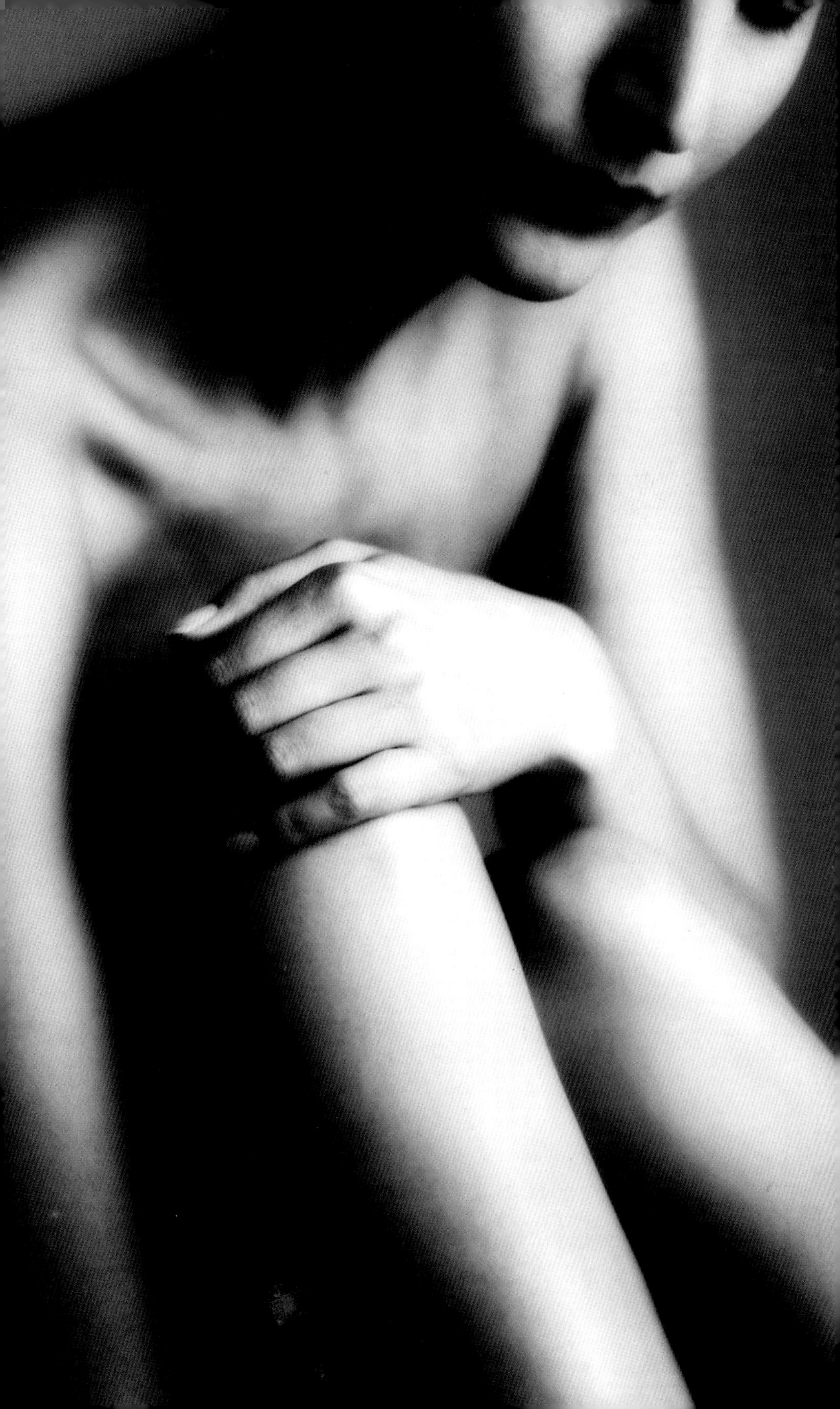

Sutra 30 Uddalika has described the gains and losses on both sides as follows:

Sutra 31 If, when living with a lover, a courtesan gets both wealth and pleasure from him, it is called a "gain on both sides".

Sutra 32 When a courtesan lives with a lover at her own expense without getting any profit out of it, and the lover even takes back what he may have formerly given her, it is called a "loss on both sides".

Sutra 33 When a courtesan is uncertain whether a new acquaintance will become attached to her, and, moreover, if he did become attached to her, whether he would give her anything, it is then called a "doubt on both sides about gains".

Sutra 34 When a courtesan is uncertain whether a new lover, courted by her at her own expense, will pay or not, and at the same time wonders if her erstwhile lover will be opposed to her going to a new lover and do her some injury on account of a grudge against her; or, if having become attached to her, he would take away angrily from her anything that he may have given to her, this is called a "doubt on both sides about loss".

Sutra 35 Babhravya has described the gains and losses on both sides as follows:

When a courtesan can get money from a man whom she may go to see, and also money from a man whom she may not go to see, this is called a "gain on both sides".

Sutra 36 When a courtesan has to incur further expense if she goes to see a man, and yet runs the risk of incurring an irremediable loss if she does not go to see him, this is called a "loss on both sides".

Sutra 37 When a courtesan is uncertain whether a particular man would give her anything on her going to see him, without incurring expense on her part, or whether on her neglecting him another man would give her something, this is called a "doubt on both sides about gain".

Sutra 38 When a courtesan is uncertain whether, on going at her own expense to see an old enemy, he would take back from her what he may have given her, or whether by her not going to see him he would cause some disaster to fall upon her, this is called a "doubt on both sides about loss".

Sutra 39 By combining the above-mentioned, the following six kinds of mixed results are produced: Gain on one side, and loss on the other.

Sutra 40 Gain on one side, and doubt of gain on the other.

Sutra 41 Gain on one side, and doubt of loss on the other.

Sutra 42 Loss on one side, and doubt of gain on the other.

Sutra 43 Loss on one side, and doubt of loss on the other.

Sutra 44 Doubt of gain on one side, and doubt of loss on the other.

Sutra 45 A courtesan, having considered all the above things and taken counsel with her friends, should act so as to acquire gain, the chances of great gain, and the warding off of any great disaster.

Sutra 46 Religious merit and pleasure should also be formed into separate combinations like those of wealth, and then all should be combined with each other, so as to form new combinations.

Sutras 47–50 When a courtesan consorts with men, she should cause each of them to give her money as well as pleasure. At particular times, such as the spring festivals, and so on, she should make her mother announce to the various men that on a certain day her daughter will remain with the man who gratifies such and such a desire of hers.

Sutra 51 When young men approach her with delight, she should think of what she may accomplish through them.

Sutra 52 The combination of gains and losses on all sides are: gain on one side, and loss on all others; loss on one side and gain on all others; gain on all sides; and loss on all sides.

Sutra 53 A courtesan should also consider doubts about gain and doubts about loss with reference to wealth, religious merit and pleasure.

Thus ends the consideration of gain, loss, attendant gains, attendant losses and doubts.

Sutra 54 The different kinds of courtesans are: a bawd, a female attendant, an unchaste woman, a dancing girl, a female artisan, a woman who has left her family, a woman living on her beauty, and, finally, a regular courtesan.

Sutra 55 All the above kinds of courtesans are acquainted with various kinds of men, and should consider the ways of getting money from them, of pleasing them, of separating themselves from them, and of reuniting with them. They should also take into consideration particular gains and losses, attendant gains and losses, and doubts in accordance with their several conditions.

Thus ends the consideration of courtesans.

Sutra 56 There are also two verses on the subject as follows:
"Men want pleasure, while women want money, and therefore this part, which deals with the means of gaining wealth, should be studied."

Sutra 57 "There are some women who seek love, and there are others who seek money; for the former the ways of love are told in previous portions of this work, while the ways of getting money, as practised by courtesans, are described in this part."

NOTES

1. In England the lower classes of courtesans walk the streets; in India and other places in the East, they sit at the windows or at the doors of their houses.
2. On the completion of a vow, a festival takes place. Some trees, such as the banyan, are invested with sacred threads, like the Brahmin's, and on the occasion of this ceremony a festival is held. In the same way, when gardens are made, and tanks or temples built, then festivities are also observed.
3. A mixture of betel nut and betel leaves.
4. The souls of men who die with their desires unfulfilled are said to go to the world of the *manes*, and not directly to the supreme spirit. (*Manes* were the souls of deceased loved ones in pagan ancient Rome – minor spirits similar to the *lares*, *genii* and *penates*.)

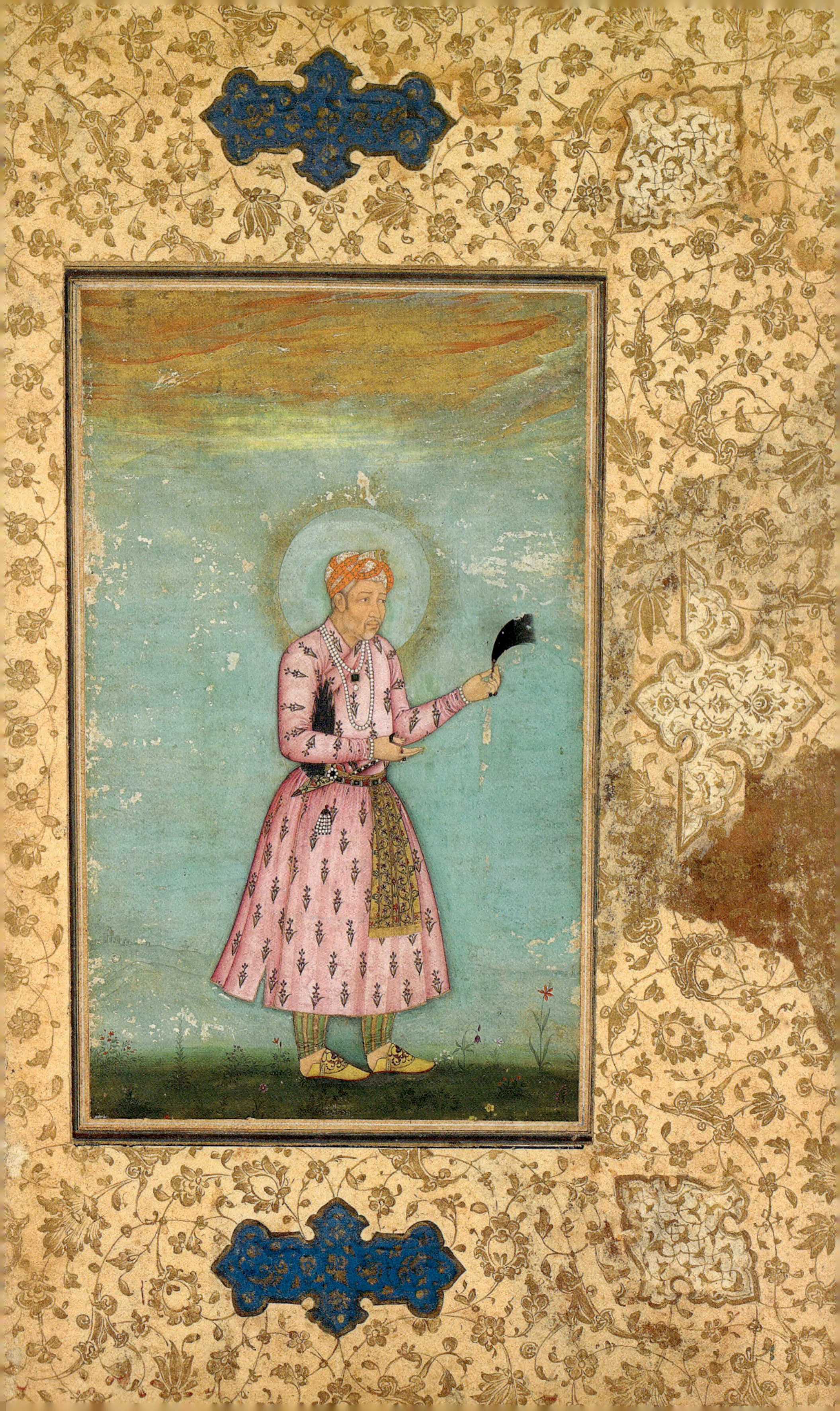

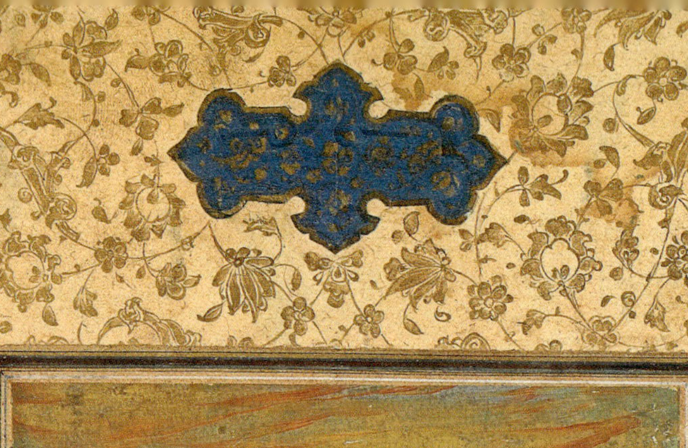

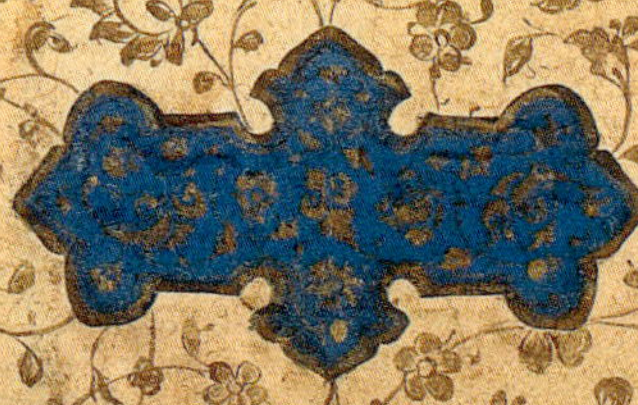

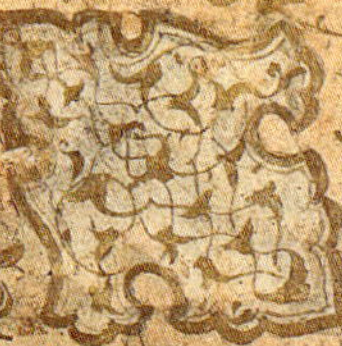

Part Seven: On Ways of Making Oneself Attractive to Others

Chapter I Personal adornment; subjugating the hearts of others; and tonic medicines

Sutra 1 When a person fails to obtain the object of his desires by any of the ways previously related, he should then have recourse to other ways of attracting others to himself.

Sutra 2 Good looks, good qualities, youth and liberality are the chief and most natural means of making a person agreeable to others. But in the absence of these a man or a woman must have resort to artificial means, or to art, and the following recipes may be found useful.

Sutra 3 An ointment made of crepe jasmine [*Tabernaemontana coronaria*], crepe ginger [*Costus speciosus*] or ginger [*Costus arabicus*], and plum [*Flacourtia cataphracta*] can be used as an unguent of adornment.

Sutras 4–5 If these plants are made into a fine powder and applied to the wick of a lamp made to burn with the oil of blue vitrol [copper sulphate], the resultant lamp black applied to the eyelashes looks lovely.

Sutra 6 Applied to the body, the oil of hogweed [*Boerhaavia diffusa*], the sariva plant, the yellow amaranth and water lily has the same effect.

Sutra 7 A black pigment from the same plants produces a similar effect.

Sutra 8 By eating powdered wild lotus [*Nelumbium speciosum*] and *Mesua ferrea* [*nagkesar*], with ghee and honey, a man becomes lovely.

Sutra 9 The above things, together with crepe jasmine [*Tabernaemontana coronaria*] and Himalayan Garcinia [*Xanthochymus pictorius*] used as an ointment, produce the same results.

Sutra 10 The eye of a peacock set in gold, and tied on the right hand or arm, makes a man lovely in the eyes of others.

Sutra 11 In the same way, if a bead made of the seed of the jujube, or of the conch shell, be enchanted by the incantations mentioned in the *Atharva Veda*, or by the incantations of those skilled in magic, and tied on the hand, it produces the same result as described above.

Sutra 12 When a female attendant reaches puberty, her master should keep her secluded, and when men ardently desire her on account of her seclusion, and on account of the difficulty of approaching her, he should then bestow her hand on such a person as may endow her with wealth and happiness.

This is a means of increasing the loveliness of a person in the eyes of others.

Sutra 13 In the same way, when the daughter of a courtesan reaches puberty, the mother should get together a lot of young men of the same age, disposition and knowledge as her daughter, and tell them that she will give her in marriage to the person who gives her presents of a particular kind.

After this the daughter should be kept in seclusion as far as possible, and the mother should give her in marriage to the man who may be ready to give her the presents agreed upon. If the mother is unable to get so much out of the man, she should show some of her own things as having been given to the daughter by the bridegroom.

Or the mother may allow her daughter to be married to the man

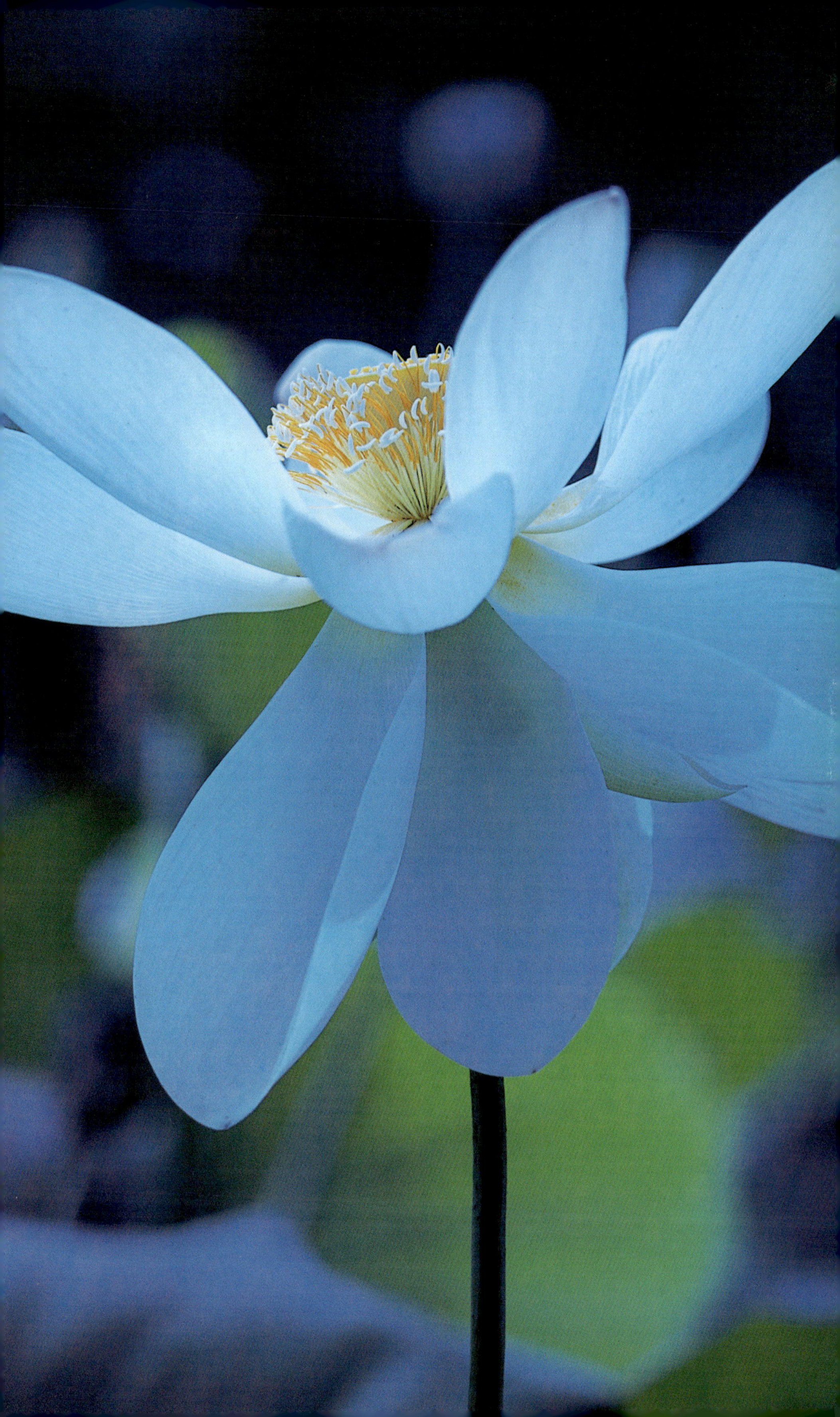

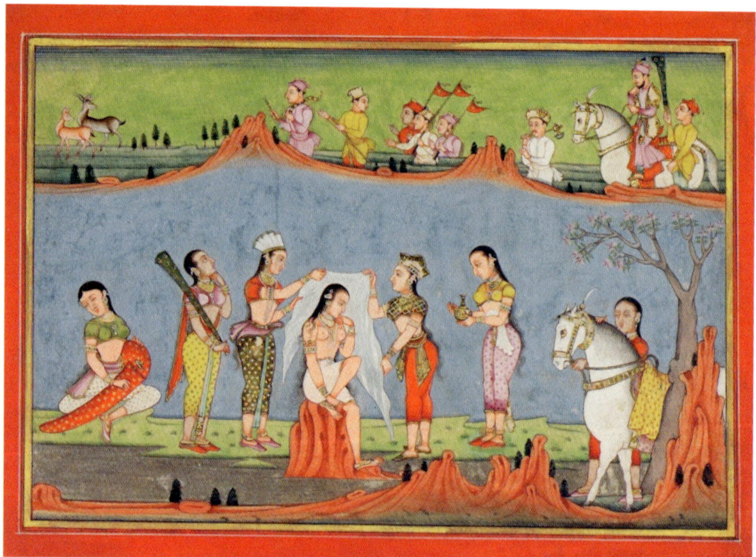

privately, as if she was ignorant of the whole affair; then, pretending that it has come to her knowledge, she may give her consent to the union.

Sutra 14 The daughter, unbeknown to her mother, should court the sons of wealthy citizens and make them attracted to her.

Sutras 15–20 For this purpose she should meet them when learning to sing, in places where music is played and at the houses of other people, and then ask of her mother, through a female friend, or servant, to be allowed to unite with the man who is most agreeable to her.[1]

Sutra 21 When the daughter of a courtesan is thus given to a man the ties of marriage should be observed for one year, and after that she may do what she likes.

Sutra 22 But even after the end of the year, when she is otherwise engaged and then invited by her first husband to come and see him, she should put aside her thought of gain, and return to him for the night.

Such is the mode of temporary marriage among courtesans, and of increasing their loveliness and their value in the eyes of others.

Sutra 23 What has been said should also be understood to apply to the daughters of dancing women.

Sutra 24 The difference is that their mothers should give them only to such persons as are likely to become useful to them in various ways.

Thus ends the ways of making oneself lovely in the eyes of others.

Sutra 25 If a man, after smearing his *lingam* with a mixture of the powders of the white thorn apple, the long pepper and the black pepper, and honey, engages in sexual union with a woman, he makes her subject to his will.

Sutra 26 The application of a mixture of leaves from the *vatodbhranta* plant, the flowers garlanding a human corpse due to be cremated, powdered bones of the peacock and of the *jivanjivaka* [pheasant] bird produces the same effect.

Sutra 27 The remains of a kite that has died a natural death, ground into powder and mixed with gooseberry [*amalaka; Phyllanthus emblica*] and honey, has the same effect.

Sutra 28 Anointing oneself with an ointment made of gooseberry has the power of subjecting women to one's will.

Sutra 29 If a man cuts the sprouts of the *vajrashnuhi* plant into small pieces and dips them into a mixture of red arsenic and sulphur, then dries them seven times and applies this powder, mixed with honey, to his *lingam*, he can subjugate a woman to his will from the moment that he has sexual union with her; or if, when burning these same sprouts at night and then looking at the smoke, he sees a golden moon behind, he will be successful with any woman.

Sutra 30 If he throws some of the powder of these same sprouts mixed with the excrement of a monkey upon a maiden, she will not be given in marriage to anybody else.

Sutras 31–33 If pieces of *vacha* [*Acorus calamus*] are dressed with mango juice and placed for six months in a hole in the trunk of the *sisu* tree [rosewood], and are then taken out, made into an ointment and applied to the *lingam*, this is said to be a means of subjugating women.

Sutra 34 If a camel bone is dipped into the juice of the *bhringraj* plant [*Eclipta prostata*] then burned, the black pigment produced should be placed in a box, also made of camel bone, and then applied together with antimony to the eyelashes with a pencil, again made of camel bone. The pigment is said to be very pure and wholesome for the eyes, and it serves as a means of subjugating others to the person who uses it.

Sutra 35 The same effect can be produced by black pigment made of the bones of hawks, vultures and peacocks.

Thus ends the ways of subjugating others to one's own will.

Now the means of increasing sexual vigour are as follows:

Sutra 36 A man obtains sexual energy by drinking milk mixed with sugar, the root of the *uchchata* plant, piper chaba and liquorice.

Sutra 37 Drinking milk mixed with sugar and with the testicle of a ram or a goat boiled in it also makes a man virile.

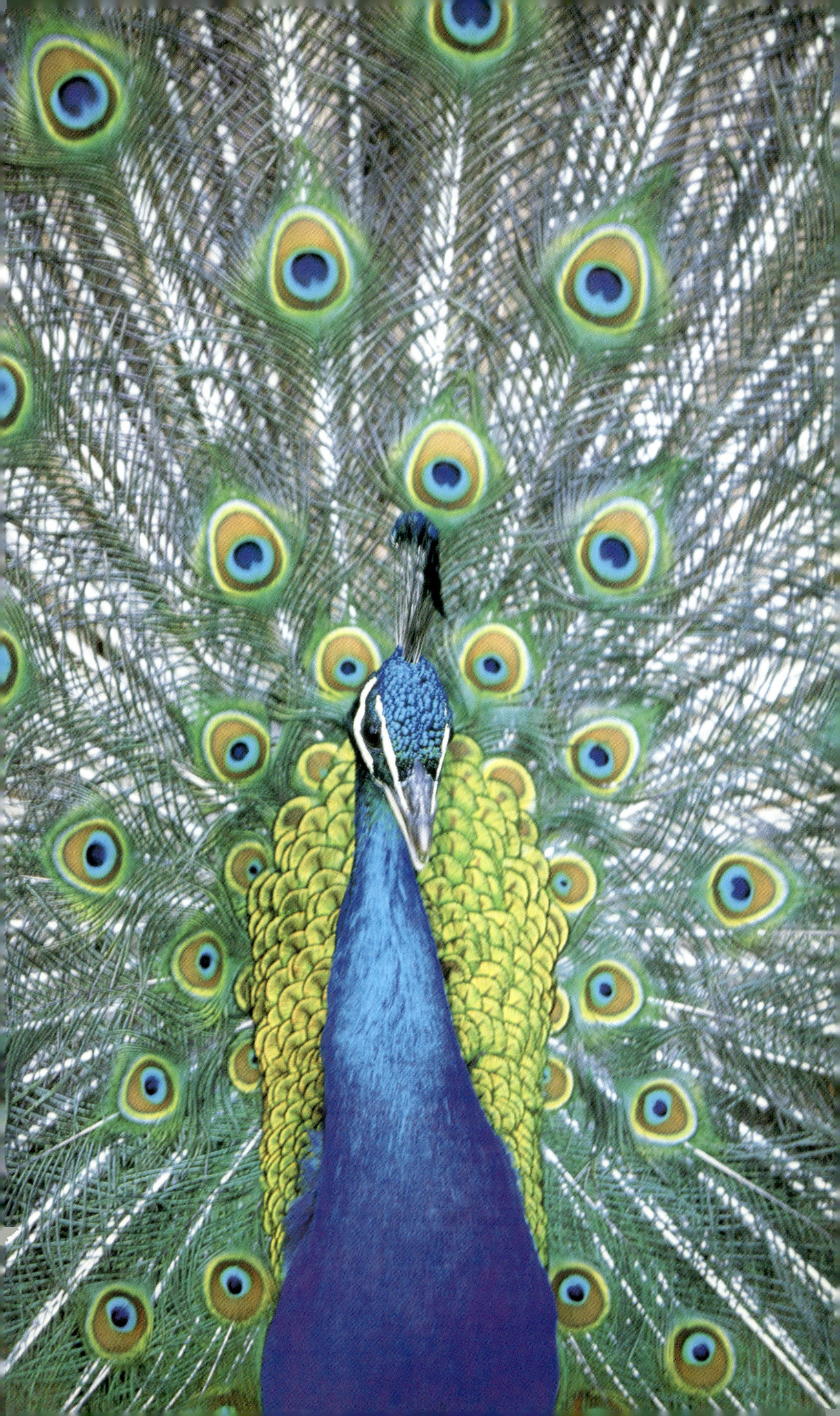

Sutra 38 Drinking the juice of sal-leaved Desmodium [*Hedysarum gangeticum*], the *kuili* and the *kshirika* plant, mixed with milk, produces the same effect.

Sutra 39 The seed of the long pepper along with those of Indian bowstring hemp [*Sansevieria roxburghiana*] and sal-leaved Desmodium, all pounded together and mixed with milk, produces a similar result.

Sutra 40 According to ancient sages, if a man pounds the seeds or roots of water chestnut [*Trapa bispinosa*], *kasurika*, tuscan jasmine and liquorice, together with *kshirakapoli* (a kind of onion), and puts the powder into milk mixed with sugar and ghee, then boils the whole mixture and drinks the paste, he will be able to enjoy many women.

Sutra 41 In the same way, if a man mixes rice with a sparrow's eggs, boils that in milk, adds to it ghee and honey, and drinks as much of it as necessary, this will produce the same effect.

Sutra 42 If a man takes the outer covering of sesamum seeds and soaks them with sparrow eggs, boils them in milk mixed with suga, ghee, the fruits of the water chestnut and *kasurika* plants, wheat flour and beans, and then drinks the composition, he is able to enjoy many women.

Sutra 43 If equal quantities of ghee, honey, sugar and liquorice are mixed together with the juice of fennel and milk this nectar-like composition is said to be holy and to provoke sexual vigour.

Sutra 44 The drinking, in spring, of a paste composed of *satawari* [*Asparagus racemosus*], the *shvadaushtra* plant, the *guduchi* plant, the long pepper and liquorice, boiled in milk, honey and ghee, is said to have the same effect as the above.

Sutra 45 Boiling in water the *satawari* and the *shvadaushtra* plants, along with the pounded fruits of *Premna spinosa*, and drinking the product is said to act in the same way.

Sutra 46 Drinking boiled ghee, or clarified butter, on a spring morning is said to be beneficial to health and strength and agreeable to the taste.

Sutras 47–48 If the powdered seed of the *shvadaushtra* plant and barley are mixed together in equal parts, and a portion of it two *pala*s [130g] in weight is eaten every morning on getting up, it has the same effect as the preceding recipe.

Sutra 49 There are also verses on the subject as follows:
"The means[2] of producing love and sexual vigour should be learned from the science of medicine, from the *veda*s, from those who are learned in the arts of magic, and from confidential relatives.

Sutra 50 No means should be tried which are doubtful in their effects, which are likely to cause injury to the body, which involve the death of animals, and which bring us into contact with impure things.

Sutra 51 Such means should only be used as are holy, acknowledged to be good, and approved of by Brahmins and friends."

Chapter II The ways of exciting desire, and miscellaneous experiments and recipes

Sutras 1–3 If a man is unable to satisfy a *hastini*, or elephant woman, he should have recourse to various means to excite her passion. At the beginning he should rub her *yoni* with his hand or fingers, and not begin to have intercourse with her until she becomes excited, or

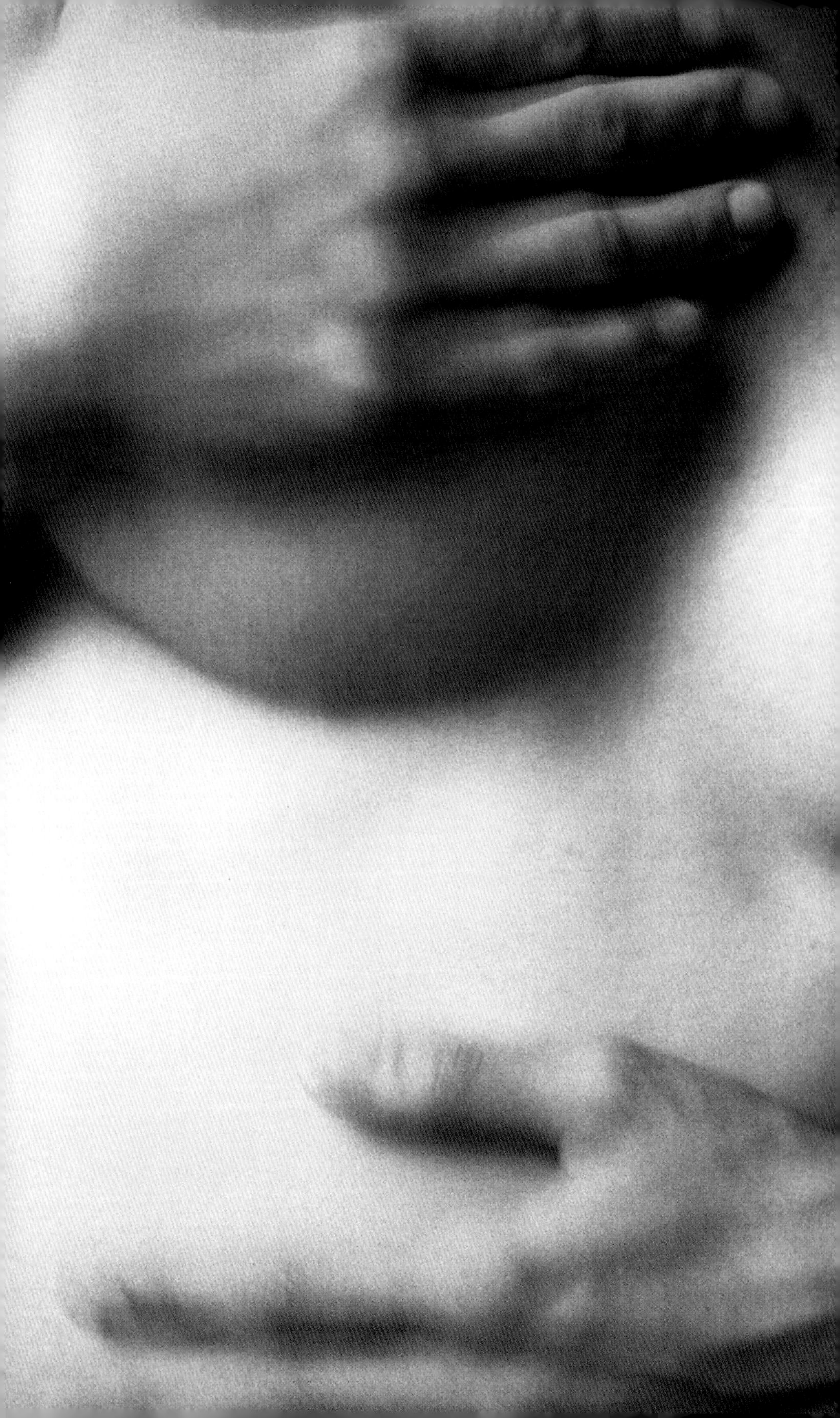

experiences pleasure. This is one way of exciting a woman.

Sutras 4–5 Or, he may make use of certain *apadravyas*, or things which are put on or around the *lingam* to supplement its length or its thickness, so as to fit it to the *yoni*.

Sutra 6 In the opinion of Babhravya, these *apadravyas* should be made of gold, silver, copper, iron, ivory, buffalo's horn, various kinds of wood, tin or lead, and should be soft, cool, provocative of sexual vigour and fitted well to serve the intended purpose.

Sutra 7 Vatsyayana, however, says that they may be made according to the natural liking of each individual.

The following are the different kinds of *apadravyas*:

Sutra 8 The "armlet" (*valaya*) should be of the same size as the *lingam*, and should have its outer surface roughly textured.

Sutra 9 The "couple" (*sanghati*) is formed of two pieces.

Sutra 10 The "bracelet" (*chudaka*) is made by joining three or more pieces until they match the required length of the *lingam*.

Sutra 11 The "single bracelet" is formed by wrapping a single wire around the *lingam*, according to its dimensions.

Sutra 12 The *kantuka* or *jalaka* is tied to the waist and is a tube open at both ends, with a hole through it, outwardly rough and studded with soft protrusions.

Sutra 13 When such a thing cannot be obtained, then use may be made of an improvised aid, perhaps using a tube made of applewood, a tubular stalk of the bottle gourd, or a reed made soft with oil and plant extracts, and tied to the waist with strings.

The above are the things that can be used in connection with or in the place of the *lingam*.

Sutras 14–15 The people of the southern regions think that true sexual pleasure cannot be obtained without perforating the *lingam*, and they therefore make a hole in it like an infant's lobes pierced for earrings.

Sutra 16 When a young man perforates his *lingam* he should pierce it with a sharp instrument, and stand in water for as long as it bleeds.

Sutra 17 At night he should engage in sexual intercourse, even with vigour, in order to clean the hole.

Sutra 18–20 After this he should continue to wash the hole with decoctions.

Sutras 21–22 He should gradually enlarge the orifice by putting into it small pieces of cane and Arctic snow [*Wrightia antidysenterica*]. It may also be washed with liquorice mixed with honey, and the size of the hole increased by using the fruit stalks of the *simapatra* plant. The hole should also be anointed with a small quantity of oil.

Sutra 23 In the hole made in the *lingam* a man may put *apadravya*s of various forms.

Sutra 24 Such as the "round", the "round on one side", the "wooden mortar", the "flower", the "armlet", the "bone of the heron", the "goad of the elephant", the "collection of eight balls", the "lock of hair", the "place where four roads meet", and other things named according to their forms and means of using them. All these *apadravyas* should be textured on the outside according to their requirements.

The ways of enlarging the *lingam* must be now related.

Sutra 25 When a man wishes to enlarge his *lingam* he should rub it with the bristles of certain insects that live in trees, and then, after rubbing it for ten nights with oils, he should again rub it with the bristles as before. By continuing to do this a swelling will be gradually produced in the *lingam*, and he should then lie on a cot and cause his *lingam* to hang down through a hole in the cot.

Sutra 26 After this he should take away all the pain from the swelling by using cool concoctions.

Sutra 27 The swelling, which is called "*suka*", lasts for life.

Sutra 28 If the *lingam* is rubbed with *ashwagandha* [*Physalis flexuosa*], the *shavara-kandaka* plant, the *jalasuka* plant, the fruit of the eggplant, the butter of a she buffalo, the *hastri-charma* plant, and the juice of the *vajrarasa* plant, a swelling lasting for one month will be produced.

Sutra 29 By rubbing it with oil boiled in the concoctions of the above things the same effect will be produced, but lasting for six months.

Sutra 30 The enlargement of the *lingam* is also effected by rubbing it or moistening it with oil boiled on a moderate fire along with the seeds of the pomegranate and the cucumber, the juices of the *valuka* plant, the *hastri-charma* plant and the eggplant.

Sutra 31 In addition to the above, other means may be learned from experienced and confidential persons.

The miscellaneous experiments and recipes are as follows:

Sutra 32 If a man mixes powdered milk hedge plant and *kantaka* plant with the excrement of a monkey and the powdered root of the *lanjalika* plant, and throws this mixture on a woman, she will not love anybody else afterwards.

Sutra 33 If a man thickens up the fruit juice of the golden shower tree [*Cassia fistula*] and the rose apple [*Eugenia jambolana*] by mixing them with powdered *soma* plant, ironweed [*Vernonia anthelmintica*], *bhringraj* [*Eclipta prostrata*] and *lohopa-jihirka*, then applies this to the *yoni* of a woman and has sexual intercourse with her, his love for her will be destroyed.

Sutra 34 The same effect is produced if a man connects with a woman who has bathed in she-buffalo buttermilk mixed with the powders of the *gopalika* and *banu-padika* plants and the yellow amaranth.

Sutra 35 An ointment made of the flowers of *kadam* [*Nauclea cadamba*], the hog plum and *jambul* [*Eugenia jambolana*], and used by a woman, causes her to be disliked by her husband.

Garlands made of the above flowers, when worn by the woman, produce the same effect.

Sutra 36 An ointment made of the fruit of the *kokilaksha* plant [*Asteracantha longifolia*] will contract the *yoni* of a *hastini*, or elephant woman, and this contraction lasts for one night.

Sutra 37 An ointment made by pounding the roots of the wild lotus [*Nelumbium speciosum*], the blue lotus and powdered *ashwagandha*

[*Physalis flexuosa*], mixed with ghee and honey, will enlarge the *yoni* of the *mrigi*, or deer woman.

Sutra 38 An ointment made of the fruit of *Emblica myrabolans*[3] soaked in the milky juice of the milk hedge plant, the *soma* plant, crown flower [*Calotropis gigantea*] and the juice of the fruit of ironweed will make the hair white.

Sutra 39 The juice of the roots of the *madayantika* plant, the yellow amaranth, the *anjanika* plant, the butterfly pea [*Clitoria ternatea*] and the *shlakshnaparin* plant will make the hair grow when used as a lotion.

Sutra 40 An ointment made by boiling the above roots in oil will make the hair black and will also gradually restore hair that has fallen out.

Sutra 41 If *lac* is saturated seven times in the sweat of a white horse's testicle and applied to a red lip, the lip will become white.

Sutra 42 The colour of the lips can be regained by means of *madayantika* and other plants mentioned above.

Sutra 43 A woman who hears a man playing on a reed pipe which has been dressed with the juices of the *bahupadika* plant, crepe jasmine, crepe ginger or ginger, *Pinus deodara*, triangular spurge [*Euphorbia antiquorum*], and the *vajra* and *kantaka* plants, becomes his slave.

Sutra 44 If food is mixed with the fruit of the thorn apple [*Datura stramonium*] it causes intoxication.

Sutra 45 If water is mixed with oil and the ashes of any kind of grass except the *kusha* grass it becomes the colour of milk.

Sutra 46 If yellow *myrabolans*, the hog plum, the *shrawana* plant and the *priyangu* plant are all pounded together and applied to iron pots, these pots become red.

Sutras 47–49 If a lamp, trimmed with oil extracted from the *shrawana* and *priyangu* plants, its wick being made of cloth and the slough of snakes, is lit and long pieces of wood are placed near it, those pieces of wood will resemble so many snakes.

Sutra 50 Drinking the milk of a white cow who has a white calf at her foot is auspicious, produces fame and prolongs life.

Sutra 51 The blessings of venerable Brahmins, well propitiated, have the same effect.

There are also some verses in conclusion:

Sutra 52 "Thus have I written in a few words the 'science of love', after reading the texts of ancient authors, and following the ways of enjoyment mentioned in them."

Sutra 53 "He who is acquainted with the true principles of this science pays regard to Dharma, Artha, Kama and to his own experiences, as well as to the teachings of others, and does not act simply on the dictates of his own desire."

Sutra 54 "As for the errors in the 'science of love' which I have mentioned on my own authority as an author, I have, immediately after mentioning them, carefully censured and prohibited them."

Sutra 55 "Just because this work mentions an act it should not be understood that it is to be undertaken; it ought to be remembered that it is the intention of this work that the rules it contains should only be acted upon in particular cases."

Sutras 56–57 "After reading and considering the works of Babhravya and other ancient sages, and thinking over the meaning of the rules given by them, the *Kama Sutra* was composed, according to the precepts of Holy Writ and for the benefit of the world, by Vatsyayana, while he was leading the life of a religious student and wholly engaged in the contemplation of the Deity."

Sutra 58 "This work is not intended to be used merely as an instrument for satisfying our desires. A person, acquainted with the true principles of this science, and who preserves his Dharma, Artha and Kama, and has regard for the practices of the people, is sure to obtain mastery over his senses."

Sutra 59 "In short, an intelligent and prudent person, attending to Dharma and Artha, and attending to Kama also, without becoming the slave of his passions, obtains success in everything that he may undertake."

NOTES

1. It is a custom of the courtesans of the East to give their daughters temporarily in marriage when they come of age, and after they have received an education in the *Kama Sutra* and other arts. Full details of this are given on page 76 of *Early Ideas*, stories collected and collated by Anaryan (W.H. Allen & Co., London, 1881).
2. From the earliest times Eastern authors have written about aphrodisiacs. The following note was taken from a translation of the *Anunga Runga*, alluded to in the Preface and Introduction of this work [see pages 7 and 11]: "Most Eastern treatises divide aphrodisiacs into two different kinds: the mechanical or natural, such as scarification, flagellation, etc.; and the medicinal or artificial. To the former belong the application of insects; all orientalists will remember the tale of the old Brahmin whose young wife insisted on him being stung again by a wasp."
3. Also often identified as *Phyllanthus emblica*, which is gooseberry, cited elsewhere here.

A Chronology of Ancient India

c.2600–1900BCE: Flowering of the Indus Valley Civilization

c.1500BCE: Aryans move into India via Afghanistan and Iraq. Texts are composed in Indo-European Vedic, including the *Rig Veda*. Beginnings of the caste system.

c.800–400BCE: The Upanishads are composed in Sanskrit

c.563–c.483BCE: Life of Siddhartha Gautama, founder of Buddhism

c.500BCE: Jainism established in northern India

c.400BCE: Vyasa composes the world's longest epic poem, the *Mahabharata*

327BCE: Alexander the Great of Macedonia invades the Indus valley

c.300BCE: The *Ramayana* is composed

c.273–232BCE: Rule of the Buddhist emperor Ashoka the Great. Maurya dynasty expands to almost all of India.

c.150BCE: Patanjali writes the *Yoga Sutras*

c.100BCE: The *Bhagavad Gita* is composed

c.50CE: Thomas, an apostle of Jesus, visits India

c.200: The Code of Manu puts down the rules of everyday life and divides Hindus into four major castes

c.250: Gupta dynasty established in northern India

c.550: Decline of Gupta Empire

c.800: Rise to prominence of Rajputs in central India and Rajasthan

c.850: Emergence of Chola power in Tamil Nadu

c.900: *Kavyaprakasha* composed

c.900–1200: *Jayamangla* composed

c.950–1050: Temple complex at Khajuraho constructed

c.997: Mahmud of Ghazni raids northern India and conquers the Punjab

c.1192: Mohammad of Ghori captures Delhi and establishes Muslim rule in India

1206: Qutub-ud-din Aibak becomes the first sultan of Delhi

c.1250: Decline of Chola dynasty

c.1500: Sikhism established by Guru Nanak Dev Ji

1498: Vasco da Gama lands at Calicut

1510: Portuguese seize Goa

1526: Babur, an Afghan ruler, establishes the Mughal dynasty in India. Flowering of Mughal art, architecture, literature and music.

1556–1605: Reign of Mughal Emperor Akbar

1600: East India Company is established

1632–53: Shah Jahan builds the Taj Mahal, a memorial to his beloved wife Mumtaz

Further Reading

Avari, Burjor. *India: The Ancient Past.* Routledge: London, 2007.

Balsam, A.L. *The Origins and Development of Classical Hinduism.* Oxford University Press: Oxford, 1991.

Bell, T. *Kalogynomia, or, The laws of female beauty: being the elementary principles of that science.* Walpole Press and J.J. Stockdale: London, 1821.

Buitenen, J.A.B. van. (Edited by Ludo Rocher.) *Studies in Indian Literature and Philosophy.* American Institute of Indian Studies and Motilal Banarsidass Publishers: New Delhi, 1988.

Burton, Richard F. and Arbuthnot, F.F. *The Ananga Ranga.* Lancer Books: New York, 1964.

Craven, Roy C. *Indian Art: A Concise History.* Thames and Hudson: London, 1997.

Daniélou, Alain. *The Hindu Temple: Deification of Eroticism.* Inner Traditions: Rochester, Vermont, 2001.

Dehejia, Harsha V. *The Flute and the Lotus: Romantic Moments in Indian Poetry and Painting.* Mapin Publishing: Ahmedabad, 2002.

Doniger, Wendy. *The Hindus: An Alternative History.* Penguin Press: London, 2009.

Drysdale, George R. *The Elements of Social Science: Physical, Sexual, and Natural Religion.* E. Truelove: London, 1877.

Harle, J.C. *The Art and Architecture of the Indian Subcontinent.* Penguin Books: London, 1986.

Keay, John. *India: A History.* HarperCollins Publishers: London, 2001.

Keith, A.B. *A History of Sanskrit Literature.* Motilal Banarsidass Publishers: New Delhi, 2007.

Mayer, Johann Jakob. *Sexual Life in Ancient India: A Study in the Comparative History of Indian Culture.* Barnes & Noble, Inc.: New York, 1953.

McConnachie, James. *The Book of Love: In Search of the Kamasutra.* Atlantic Books: London, 2007.

Mitter, Partha. *Indian Art.* Oxford University Press: Oxford, 2001.

The New Cambridge History of India. Volumes 1–8. Cambridge University Press: Cambridge, 1987–2005.

Ram-Prasad, Chakravarthi. *India: Life, Myth & Art.* Duncan Baird Publishers: London, 2006.

Renou, Louis. (Translated by Philip Spratt.) *The Civilization in Ancient India.* South Asia Books: London, 1997.

Rice, Edward. *Captain Sir Richard Francis Burton: A Biography.* Da Capo Press: Cambridge, Massachusetts, 2008.

Roy, Kumkum. *The A to Z of Ancient India.* The Scarecrow Press: Lanham, Maryland, 2010.

Thapar, Romila. *Early India: From the Origins to AD 1300.* University of California Press: Berkeley, California, 2003.

Thomas, P. *Kama Kalpa or The Hindu Ritual of Love.* D.B. Taraporevala Sons: Bombay, 1959.

Vatsayana. (Translated by S.C. Upadhyaya.) *The Kama Sutra: The Hindu Art of Love.* Watkins Publishing: London, 2004.

Waterstone, Richard. *India: The Cultural Companion.* Duncan Baird Publishers: London, 2002.

Winternitz, Maurice. *History of Indian Literature.* Motilal Banarsidass Publishers: New Delhi, 1999.

Index

Acknowledgments and Picture Credits

The publisher would like to thank the following people, museums and photographic libraries for permission to reproduce their material. Any errors or omissions are entirely unintentional and the publisher will, if informed, make amendments in future editions of this book:

AA The Art Archive, London; **BAL** The Bridgeman Art Library, London; **V&A Images** V&A Images, Victoria & Albert Museum, London; **WFA** Werner Forman Archive, London

Page 1 Inscribed stela with the *yakshi* Ambika, © The Trustees of the British Museum; **2** *Radha and Krishna embrace in a grove of flowering trees*, c.1780, V&A/ The Stapleton Collection/BAL; **6** Nude couple, Paul D. Van Hoy II/Photolibrary.com; **14–15** Woman's body, Edvard March/Corbis; **16** *Radha and Krishna in a wooded landscape*, Rajasthan, India, early 19th century, © V&A Images; **21** Star map, entitled *Jewel of Essence of All Sciences*, shows eastern and western hemispheres with classical constellations painted in Indian style, Sanskrit manuscript, India, c. 1840, British Library/AA; **24** Woman with henna-tattooed hands, Luca Tettoni/ Corbis; **29** *Radha and Krishna*, from a Baramasa, India. Detail from one page of a series of eight paintings bound in an album. The series are from a "Baramasa" set or "Songs of the seasons", providing visual imagery for Baramasa poetry. The main theme is that of *nayakas*' and *nayikas*' (lovers) love in union and in separation and their relationship with the months of the year. © The Trustees of the British Museum; **32** *Three women with fireworks*, India, Mughal, 1640, WFA/Gulistan Imperial Library, Teheran; **35** Young couple hugging, Arkadius Kozera/ Imagebroker/Alamy; **40** Erotic sculpture at Khajuraho temple, Madhya Pradesh, India, Chris Caldicott/Axiom Photographic Agency; **44** Rajasthani painting of embracing lovers, c.1750, Bettmann/Corbis; **46** *Two Women Approach to do Siva Puja* (opaque w/c, silver & gold on paper), from a Ragamala series, from Bahu-Jammu area, Punjab Hills, c.1700–1710, Museum of Fine Arts, Boston, Massachusetts, USA/Ross-Coomaraswamy Collection/BAL; **53** Couple embracing, Paul D. Van Hoy II/Photolibrary.com; **56** *The private pleasure of Prince Jahandar, son of Jahangir*, by Abdul Hamid, Bikaner, Rajasthan, Rajput School, c.1678–98 Fitzwilliam Museum, University of Cambridge/BAL; **61** *Vajrasattva*, also known as Vajradhara, the Supreme Buddha, identified by his hands which are held in the Vajrahumkara mudra, a thunderbolt in each. He sits in *yab-yum* with the Supreme

Wisdom Visvatara. Buddhist, 18th century, WFA/Philip Goldman Collection; **64** Album painting. The faithful of the cult of Tantra regarded sexual intercourse as the essential rite of initiation enabling them to accede to knowledge. The two principles, Shiva (male) and Shakti (his wisdom, embodied by the female), merged in the couple and transcended the sexual embrace. India, Hindu, late 18th/early 19th century, WFA/Private collection; **69** Woman kissing man's neck, Getty Images/Stone Collection; **74** *The private pleasure of the brother of Raja Bhar Mal.* The couple make love on a bed in a garden, Mughal buildings stand out against a star-lit sky, a crescent moon hangs over some trees, by Manohar, Bikaner, Rajasthan, Rajput School, c.1678–98, Fitzwilliam Museum, University of Cambridge/BAL; **77** Naked couple embracing, Andreas Heumann/Getty Images; **80** Bamboo, Marie Hickman/Corbis; **85** Couple making love, showing the proper posture for a *hastini* woman and an *ashva* man, by Govardhan, Bikaner, Rajasthan, Rajput School, c.1678–98, Fitzwilliam Museum, University of Cambridge/BAL; **88** Naked couple, Alamy Images; **93** Flower, Mary Ellen Baker/Photolibrary.com; **96** *A lover holding two champaka garlands reluctantly leaves his sleeping lady. Lalita Ragini* from a series of Ragamalas, Hyderabad, India, Hindu, 1770–80, WFA/India Office Library, London; **101** Woman's body, Edvard March/Corbis; **104** *Girl holding cup and flask*, from the Large Clive Album, Deccan, India, 18th century, © V&A Images; **106** Three gold *mohur* coins depicting the Zodiac signs Pisces (**left**), Leo (**centre**) and Libra (**right**), minted c.1617–24 under Mughal Emperor Jahangir (reigned 1608–27), India, AA; **109** *The marriage of Rama and his brothers* from the "Sangri Ramayana", Kulu-Mandi, Himachal Pradesh, Pahari School, 1760–65, National Museum of India, New Delhi, India/BAL; **114** Naked couple embracing, Trinette Reed/Getty Images; **117** Painted wooden elephant, India, © V&A Images; **120** *Radha and Krishna seated in a grove*, possibly made by Kulu, Punjab Hills, 1790, © V&A Images; **123** Tea plantation, Kerala, India, Michele Falzone/Getty Images; **125** Naked couple, Barnaby Hall/Getty Images; **128** Inlaid work with semiprecious stones using *pietra dura* technique, detail: ornamental field with floral patterns. Cenotaph of Shah Jahan inside the Taj Mahal mausoleum, Agra, Uttar Pradesh, India, erected 1632–53 under the Mughal emperor Shah Jahan in memory of his favourite wife Mumtaz Mahal, Alexey Fateev/Shutterstock image; **134** One side of a jewel casket painted by Rahim Deccani. The scene tells part of a story from the Hindu tradition, possibly the myth of Rama and Sita. Deccan, India, Hindu. c.1660, WFA/V&A Museum; **137** Two flowers floating on water, Alexander Benz/Corbis; **139** Nose ornament (*bulak*), c.1880, © V&A Images; **142** Silk, satin-weave cloth embroidered with silk yarn in chain stitch, © V&A Images; **147** Hands on sleeping woman, Paul Vozdic/Getty Images; **150** *Ladies celebrating the Holi Festival,* gouache on paper, c.1788, © V&A Images/P. C. Manuk and Miss G. M. Coles, bequest through the Art Fund; **154** Illustration of an episode from the *Bhagavad Purana*. The style places the illustration with the Mewar School of Rajasthani painting. Krishna is bathing with the *gopi*s (the wives and daughters of the cowherds) and the cowherds. Rajasthan, India, Hindu, late 18th century, WFA/ Prince of Wales Museum of Western India, Bombay; **157** Back of young woman, James Darell/Getty Images; **160** Indian miniature painting, Jaipur, Frédéric Soltan/ Corbis; **167** Erotic sculptures of Khajuraho, India, DC Premiumstock/Alamy; **170** Naked reclining woman, Mamad Mossadegh/Getty Images; **175** Detail of a palace wall-hanging depicting the legend of Krishna. Here the *gopi*s (wives and daughters of the cowherds) are shown talking among themselves. Krishna's favourite among them was Radha. India, Hindu, 19th century, WFA/Philip Goldman Collection; **178** Dahlia, David Roseburg/Corbis; **183** Ooty Lake, Kerala, India, Michele Falzone/Getty Images; **186** Young couple embracing, Scott Cunningham/ Getty Images; **191** *Ragini Varari* from a series of Ragamalas. The heroine accompanied by a servant rests under a canopy. Her pose expresses the theme of sensual love and the dish and coffee pots symbolize the *yoni* and *lingam* respectively. Rajasthan, India, Hindu, 18th century, WFA/National Gallery, Prague; **194** A prince smoking, 17th century, British Library/Photolibrary.com; **200** *As Passion Took Over*, page from a dispersed series of the *Gita Govinda* ("Song of the Dark Lord") of Jayadeva, made in Kangra or Guler, Himachal Pradesh, India, c.1775–80, Philadelphia Museum of Art Alvin O. Bellak Collection, 2004; **204** *The Hindu God-Hero Kama*, Jaipur, Rajasthan, India, 18th century, © V&A Images; **209** *Radha in conversation with elderly confidante*, c.1820–25, © V&A Images; **212** Naked couple in passionate embrace, Mark Harris/Getty Images; **217** Textile, furnishing or dress material. Cotton embroidered with silk thread. Gujarat, India, early 18th century, © V&A Images; **225** *Lovers at Daybreak*, illustration of the musical mode "Raga Vibhasa", gouache with silver and gold on paper, northern Deccan or southern Rajasthan, Indian School, c.1675, © Ashmolean Museum, University of Oxford/BAL **228** Poppy, David Roseburg/Corbis; **233** Two women seated in a pavilion on a terrace with a lake in the background. One is singing and the other is beating a drum. Painting, Rajasthan, mid-19th century, © V&A Images; **236** Hair ornament. Gold, with silver back, pin and interior, 19th century, © V&A Images; **241** Naked woman, Christopher Thomas/Getty Images; **246** Portrait of Emperor Akbar (?), Thierry Olliver/RMN; **249** Blue lotus flower, Tadayuki Naitoh/Getty Images; **250** *A princess bathing watched by a prince*, w/c on paper, eastern Deccan, c.1780, © V&A Images; **253** Peacock, Frank Lukasseck/ Corbis; **256** Hands on a woman's body, Visum Foto GmbH/Alamy.

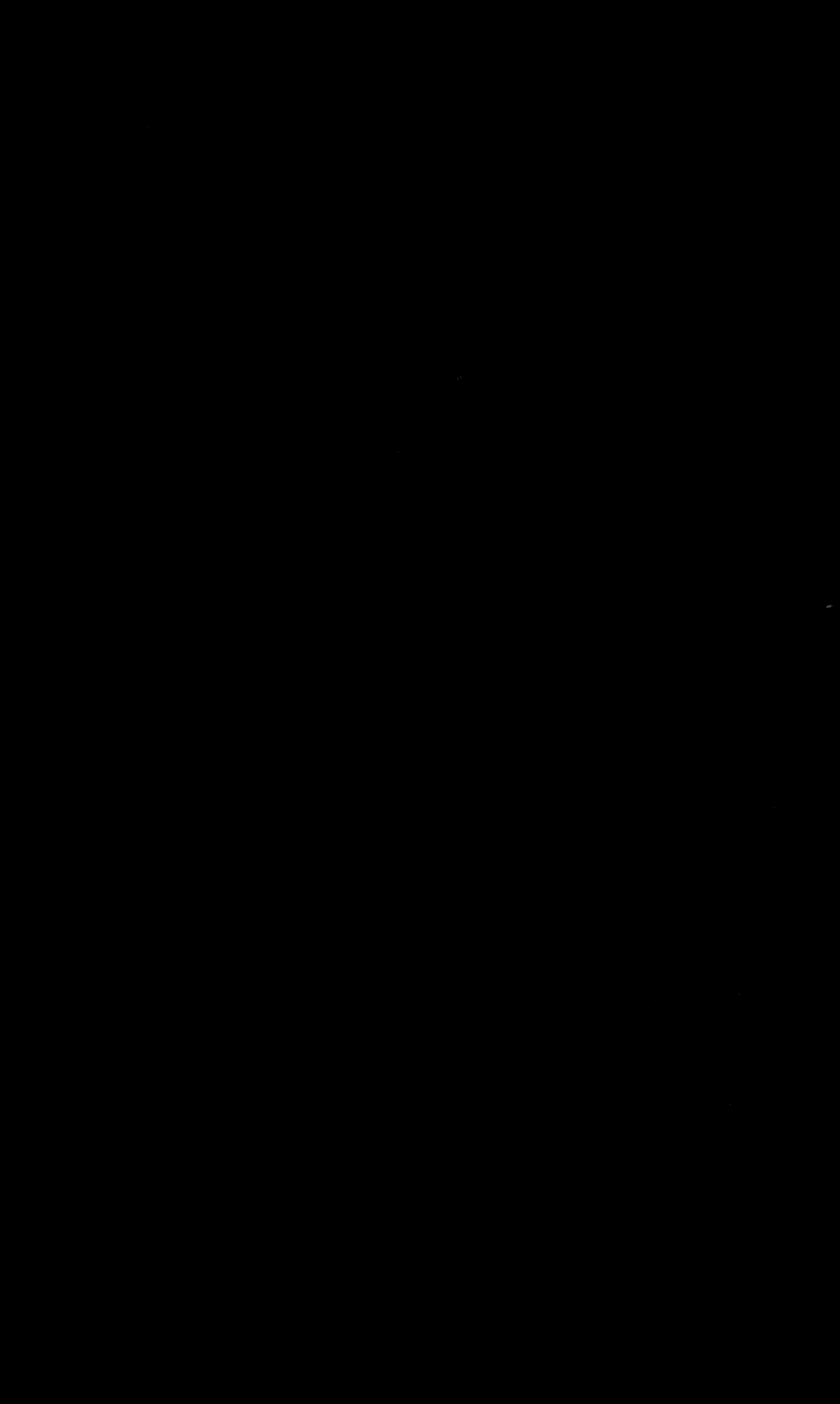

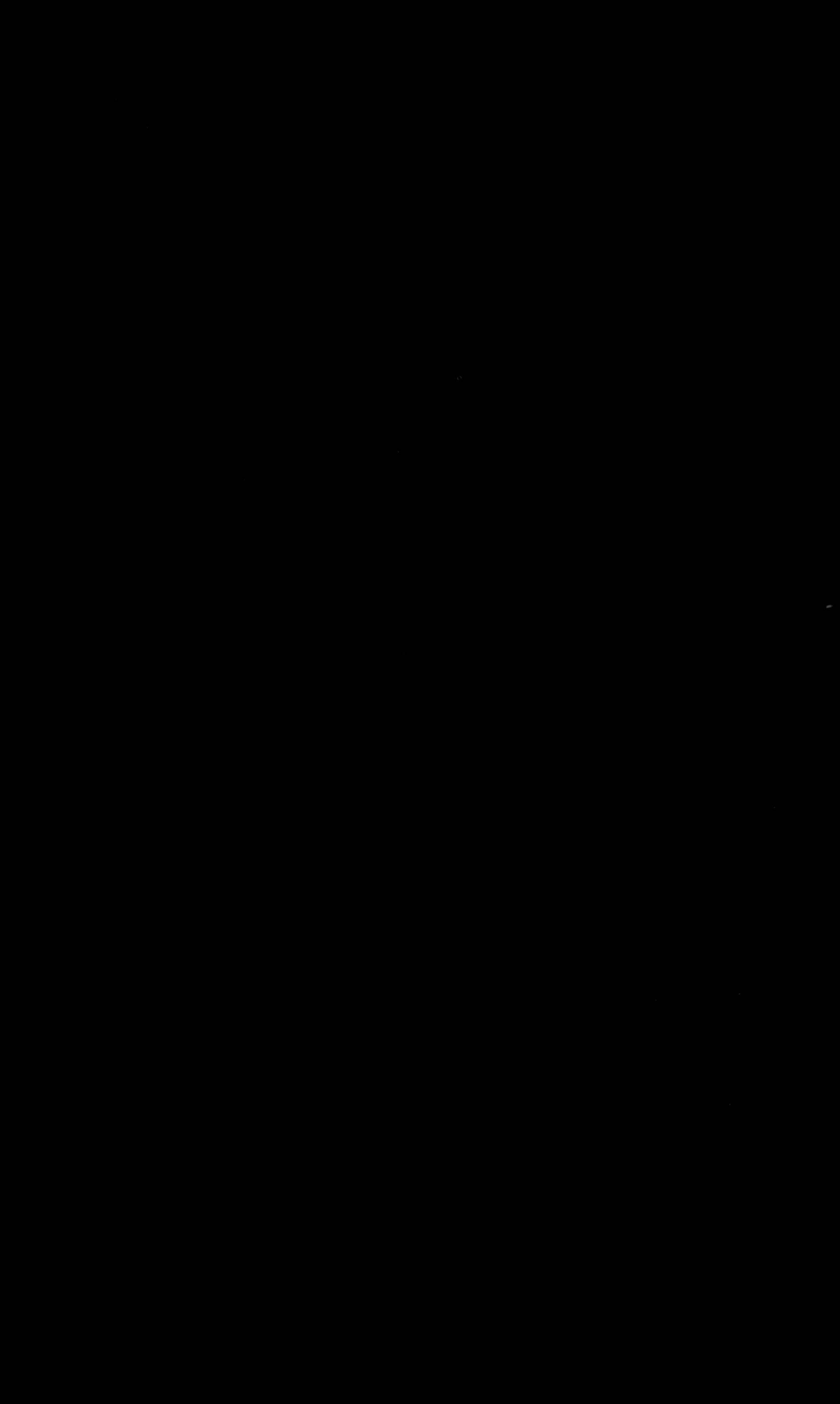